Therapist as Priest

Thanksgiving 08

To Joe —

With gratitude
for your companionship
along the way.

Prayers + Blessings for

you + yours —

Don

Therapist
as
Priest

The Spiritual Dimensions
of a Therapeutic Relationship

Donald F. Schwab

Cloverdale Books

South Bend

Therapist as Priest: The Spiritual Dimensions of a
Therapeutic Relationship

Donald F. Schwab

Published by
Cloverdale Books
An Imprint of Cloverdale Corporation
South Bend, Indiana 46601

www.CloverdaleBooks.com

Library of Congress Cataloging-in-Publication Data

Schwab, Donald Francis.
  Therapist as priest : the spiritual dimensions of a therapeutic relationship /
Donald Francis Schwab.
     p. ; cm.
  Includes bibliographical references.
  Summary: "Professional therapists working from either secular or religious
orientations are invited by this book to understand, recognize and utilize the
spiritual dimensions of a therapeutic relationship without compromising either
the science of their craft or the religious sensibilities of those who seek their
help"--Provided by publisher.
  ISBN-13: 978-1-929569-32-8 (pbk.)
  ISBN-10: 1-929569-32-7 (pbk.)
  1. Psychotherapy--Religious aspects. 2. Spirituality--Health aspects. 3.
Pastoral care. I. Title.
  [DNLM: 1. Pastoral Care--methods. 2. Religion and Medicine. 3. Spirituality.
WM 61 S398t 2007]

  RC489.S676S39 2007
  616.89'14--dc22

                                              2007019991

Printed in the United States of America
on recycled paper made from 100% post-consumer waste

Contents

Foreword

I have the good fortune in the *afternoon* of my life to reflect on the many chapters of earlier years without a moment's regret. Along with hard working parents doing their best with the resources given them, five siblings and their beautiful families, I have been immensely blessed in those who by their vocations, their knowledge and their wisdom have taught, supervised and guided me without having to make me into their own image and likeness. I count this as a blessing because of the good example it provided early on of what it means to be a spiritually-grounded guide.

These adults seemed to sense that we could all avail ourselves of another, deeper, more mysterious yet certain gift that comes from the *Holy One* alone. Call it *grace*, as they often did. That Holy Other, *God* by any name, was often invoked in their many forms of prayer. These men and women could as readily share their insights as they could candidly speak their doubt. Anselm's permission to have a *faith seeking understanding* marks so many of those who have shadowed me in the *morning years*, the *transition times*, and the days unfolding in the *here and now*. Firm in a pivotal kind of faith, these were courageous thinkers, learners and teachers. I remember and think of them as strong enough to listen with sincere interest to other sources of wisdom and insight; their lives seemed to be full, yet never complete or complacent. They managed somehow not to get *saved* in the way I experience so many people of *faith* being mired today in a kind of separatist, exclusive club which, as my favorite bumper sticker says, I believe is *neither religious [nor] right.*

Seminary rectors Rev. Drs. Joseph P. Brennan and the late + Joseph L. Hogan deserve recognition. They have my gratitude for being leaders of integrity, for providing personal spiritual growth and a vision for the future. Their educational, pastoral and spiritual leadership was exemplary not only in my early years of professional training, but critical to our local faith community as it struggled to adapt to changing times. I think, too, of Jim Marvin, a man who loved both God and people; the one who mentored and befriended me after the seminary programs launched me into parish work. As my first pastor, and like my year with [the late] Ed Steinkirchner before him, his support and example of keeping a balance in ministry between both hard work and living one's life sustains me still these many years later. [This very search for *balance* between life and work, however noble the work, brings many seekers in ministry and the human services to the doors of those who share my privilege of doing therapeutic work.] Other brothers and sisters during my priestly years -- too many to mention – kept faith, hope and fun alive along the way.

For these treasured friends, colleagues and mentors, I believe *learning* was a passion, and not just for knowledge and the success it might bring. Theirs was a hunger for *wisdom* in the ways of both God and humankind. They were, on balance, people of integrity who genuinely sought to integrate what they believed into the kind of life they led. Struggles and their clay-footed humanity were also evident, especially in later years as we moved closer to *big brother and sister*, more collegial, roles beyond those of professor-mentor and student. Today, I might think of them as open, *open systems* even, rather than just good men and good women of ever increasing knowledge and faith. It is this kind of person that I have, almost by an early-formed hunger and pursuit, surrounded myself in these later years – my *afternoon*.

Along the way, and touching only briefly on a few significant *passages* and the people who helped me navigate them, I found myself wanting to explore studies and experience work settings that eventually took me beyond the pale of ministry as priest within the Roman Catholic church. Helping me explore and understand my restlessness prior to my actual departure from ordained ministry was Dr. Richard Arnold, a clinical psychologist who gained not only my trust, but access to a carefully guarded soul. At some point, I became aware of his being Jewish, and it mattered to me as much as the polyester sheen to his clothes. Our discussions, including my *spiritual angst* concerning *call* and *vocation*, made no scary dents in his psychological training. He listened and he cared; he interpreted when helpful and called me on *my stuff* when I needed it. I am in his debt for those years and beyond.

Those who have had the chance to work with such well trained, insightful and caring professionals in the therapeutic arts and sciences know from experience that spiritual growth, when also desired, bears no necessary conflict with the scientific. The pietistic posturing of those needing to keep alive artificial separations between the metaphorical truths of religious experience and the empirical data of science seem to fear an assault on their own coveted notions of God. That kind of focused, defensive energy – allegedly spent in the cause of *truth* -- risks our failure to recognize the *Holy One's* initiative beyond personal safety zones of the *sacred*.

In one's inner work, *honesty* plays as key a role as *willingness*. Spiritual classics spoke of *surrender* long before *self- help* groups arose among us in such numbers and began to take such classic themes to themselves. The traditions of spirituality which emphasize *kenosis*, or *emptying out* [Gk.], have long taught that one cannot be filled with *self* and expect to have room for the *Holy One* and her *still small voice*. As painful as it was to have to look at the legacy of growing up in an often chaotic home where one parent was gripped with the deadly illness of alcoholism, there came a time to face that personal legacy as well. I draw attention here to this piece of my story not only out of gratitude for another caring colleague and group of professionals, but because of the large number in ministry and human services whose early life has been similarly marked by such dysfunction. For his skill, training, wisdom and guidance, I am thankful to Mr. Chuck Montante – another in a series of God-given guides whose spiritual core and professional training converged at a time when grace found me ready and willing.

I must also mention my Bishop, Matthew H. Clark. Along with brothers and sisters in the diocese where I ministered, his counsel and support was what a professional mentor and authority figure should be. A former spiritual director himself, he was empathetic, challenging, respectful of my choices and yet cautiously liberating. I mention the notion of *caution* as I write and feel my way through this reflective piece of my past. For can anyone really know what the will of God is for another when it is so hard for each of us to know it for ourselves? Don't we go, in our best moments, by prayerful discernment and our best lights? Isn't the path often one that has no certain map, never mind a guarantee of any sort? Cautious, respectful support is what I heard, and what I felt, from my bishop – another man within the ennobled *professions* whose fundamental belief was expressed to me in the humble posture of a person who himself clearly desired to do and speak healing words not simply his own: *If this [departure from ministry] is truly for your ultimate good and human freedom, it can only come from God.* Such a spiritual stance, I submit, betrays the potential for our best and most humble, human and spiritual selves as we seek to offer what wisdom, guidance and support we have as *companions* in an ultimately mysterious, yet graced, journey.

Finally, and most especially among all those who have walked with me during the intertwining path of being healed and becoming healer – as well as during the long months of crafting this work – I thank the person who most beautifully and consistently gives me glimpses of the face of God. A leader herself, a *teacher of teachers*, my wife Carole is a dedicated professional in whose orbit of love and generosity I am privileged to live and attend to my work. Her unconditional love and steady companionship – augmented not a little by our faithful Labradors – is a precious gift indeed. I am most especially humbled by this unexpected gift in my life path, the turn of events and the graced opportunity that finds me living and sharing my life with a soul friend and life companion.

If I am in the afternoon of my life, my friend and mentor, Dr. D. Wilson ["Bill"] Hess can be said to be in his twilight. Still strong, vibrant, growing and filled with a thirst for good spiritual nourishment, this man, now in his eighth decade, continues to teach so many about so much. As my primary editor and guide for this work, his red pen trimmed dozens of pages from it. In doing so, he claims to this day that it was still …*only several sentences*. I thank him not only for parsing what he commonly referred to as *the deadwood* in my manuscript, but for highlighting what is indeed most important in all of life.

To all mentioned and the many not, to clients who teach me daily about the value of the *search* and the God who guides both of us, to friends and family with me still and those who coach me from their place of light, I am, and hope to be always, a grateful and still hungry, learning and still guided, broken and still blessed companion on this common journey of ours.

Donald F. Schwab
1 April 2007

Preface

As mentioned briefly in the Forward, my current work as counselor and consultant follows significant years of training and practice as an ordained minister in a main line church. This book is not about *leaving ministry*. If anything, it may subtly argue that we never *leave anything* [or anyone] that has shaped us. So it is that I cannot consider the place of spirituality in any therapeutic relationship without drawing from the rich experiences of those privileged years. Before taking up the subject of this book, allow me to reflect on a major shift in the context of my life, including the framework of my professional endeavors, which not only significantly informs this work but compels me to write.

My journey includes a major transition from active ministry as a Roman Catholic priest to that of counselor and workplace consultant within several *secular* settings. An autobiography is neither the purpose nor the focus of this book. In the first words of the popular book *The Purpose Driven Life*, I heartily agree with author Rick Warren that *It's not about me!* Yet a glimpse of my experience as both ordained priest in a specifically *religious*, denominational setting and, later, as counselor/consultant, apart from any specifically religious settings, created the passion and inspired plans for this study.

Being a professional is not something one accomplishes on his own. Whether educational, medical, legal or religious/spiritual responsibilities are assumed for one's *work*, faculties which prepare these individuals also have standards which must be met before recognition, titles and licenses to practice are awarded. In fact, many of the professions, including those named above, require not only a specified course of academic study and supervision. They also require further periods of mentoring before one is approved for self-supervised, independent practice.

Even before such modern, more formal programs of preparation emerged, disciples attached themselves to one or more practitioners within their chosen profession or trade. The term *journeyman* remains even today and reminds us of earlier, less formal, systems of passing on both specialized theoretical knowledge and practical skills. While it is not my purpose to examine in any detail these *rites of passage* as part of professional training and practice, the impact of early models are selectively present in many current professional preparation programs.

Among those areas of service considered to be *professional* are two in which I have academic and practice credentials: ministry as ordained priest, and therapeutic work as professional counselor and consultant.

I was ordained as priestly minister within the Roman Catholic tradition in 1973 after some thirteen years of seminary preparation and study. In 1994 I received my first New York State credential in counseling. Whether the work of fate, or, as I would like to believe, the guidance of a gracious God and those who mentored me, I now find the chronological order of my life and training turned upside down. As Jung might express it, the *morning* of my life as priest has given way to its *afternoon* as a more secular, general *healer*. Twilight neither forgets nor happens without the dawn.

I will argue that any and all who seek to guide others to a fuller experience of freedom and growth as humans [made *imago dei*] as counselor, therapist or guide can, through both self-awareness and proper practice, avail themselves of that which is fundamentally spiritual *both in and among us*. It is this experience, a personal one -- phenomenological if you will -- combined with my

academic work and research, which leads me now to frame
my work as counselor/therapist within a spiritual context.
In doing so and advancing this thesis, I propose that those
who have chosen any specific secular context as the
professional setting for therapeutic work may also
consciously pay attention to the spiritual dimensions
inherent in that work. From this perspective, *healing*,
recognized or not, regains its ancient priestly roots.

My personal experience has led me to an evolving
understanding of the multi-faceted context in any
therapeutic relationship – in this case, a therapist or
counselor whose earlier spiritual orientation was informed
by religious training. I value and embrace the experience of
priestly formation and ministerial practice in a religious
setting. Far from presenting a conflict in my work as a
canonically inactive priest who currently practices as
counselor in a secular setting, the *afternoon* of my life relies
significantly on the *morning*.

It has been the long journey in company with mentors
and ongoing academic pursuits that has sustained my
interest and motivated me to seek a more formal academic
framework in which to ground my experience. Herein lays
the rationale for a personal preface.

This thesis highlights and defends what has
experientially informed my life and my professional
practice. Both chapters of my life, if you will, unfold
implicitly and explicitly in these pages. My course of study
at the Graduate Theological Foundation in the Pastoral
Psychology tract has challenged me to articulate within an
academic framework my professional experience as it
continued to unfold in tandem. As such, studies pursued
during my earlier seminary training, my work in the 1980's
culminating in the Doctor of Ministry degree and this
current, long term, project have substantiated what I now
present in this book. I understand a therapeutic
relationship with another person, community or group to
be fundamentally spiritual. Specific training or professional

context notwithstanding, any therapist or counselor has the choice to consciously apply a spiritual orientation to the therapeutic endeavor without compromising professional identity or practice methodologies.

This paper will acknowledge early on what is obvious and needs no defense. Anyone trained in Psychology/Psychiatry, Social Work or Counseling with a view to working therapeutically with others can do precisely that within a purely secular, scientific, clinically-based setting. A teacher may teach, and teach both well and responsibly, using those models of education and human development appropriate to their field. Legal professionals may avail themselves of the preparation and case examples which have accrued to their canon or corpus. Physicians need not necessarily look beyond skills, knowledge and health care delivery experience acquired during training in order to practice and dispense medicine responsibly. Professional therapists and counselors may validly operate out of a discipline that relies heavily, if not solely, on treatment strategies based on correct diagnoses.

Any of the above may exercise their profession and apply their learned craft out of either a personal faith context, or as a purist carefully guarding against any non-empirical influence or personal bias not established within their particular *case histories or canons*. It is my view that a *healer*, by any name or title, has a particularly deep spiritual well from which to draw, and one that is supported by a lengthy tradition found in both specifically spiritual as well as general, more secular, language and descriptions. The water of this well clearly flows from, and across, the deep veins of the world's religions and spiritual traditions.

Philosophical inquiry placed side by side with the social sciences can provide not only substantive insight into one's fundamental Identity as healer, but also guidance and sustenance for the privileged place healers are given in the lives of individuals and communities. As such, they naturally invite practitioners of healing to call upon resources often not mentioned or named in formal programs of preparations. Neither does such an appeal in any way negate necessary, required systems of training and knowledge. Once again, my experience *and* study have demonstrated that both are foundational.

Returning to the four, more *classic* professions mentioned earlier, and having acknowledged that at least three of the four are able to *stand alone* quite comfortably as standard practice in secular ministrations [Education, Law/Politics, Medicine], the work of *healing* not only begs the question of a *vocation* understood as *sacred* in character – and thus loom larger than tighter definitions of a profession – but, in my view, often relies explicitly on the other three to fully accomplish their professional endeavors. For even if we leave aside some of the subcategories of therapeutic, healing disciplines bearing witness to this fact [e.g., psycho-educational approaches et. al.], can there be any doubt that a person's or community's movement toward health often involves new understandings [education], an infusion of order [law/politics] or collaboration in physical treatments [medicine]?

Throughout this work I will be using the generic term *therapist* in reference to the role of healer. Specifically, this term will usually reference professionals commonly associated with the healing of one's emotional or psychological pain. When necessary to connote associations within either a broader, or more narrow, context, I will rely on both the context of the sentence, as well as the specific subject matter at hand [including chapter foci] in order to make clear the nuanced connections being dealt with at the time, e.g. therapist as priest; counselor [therapist] – client relationship; therapist-healer as professional etc. As an umbrella term to be used with greater specificity at each point of discussion, *therapeutic work*, then, connotes, and for our purposes points to, professional roles and services associated with those in the *healing professions.*

As a person and a professional, I have experienced directly a melding of the psychological and spiritual disciplines as my life, and my life's work [*vocation*], has gradually moved from the specifically religio-spiritual framework of church ministry to the more general, secular, context of counseling and consulting. Once again citing Jung's analogy, my *afternoon* of life and my life's work as healer remained ever more informed and guided by that which I was taught, learned and experienced within the similarly privileged, professional *morning years* of priestly ministry.

Introduction

The title of this work, *Therapist as Priest: The Spiritual Foundations of a Therapeutic Relationship* identifies the two areas to be explored in this book: the synthesis of a life as priest with later responsibilities as a therapist. I have described how my experiences and successive periods of training have influenced and shaped the use of various disciplines in my work settings along the way: Pastoral Theology, [Family] Systems Theory, Faith Development, Hospital Intervention work, Adult Development Psychology, work in Chemical Dependency settings et. al. These experiences, as well as my education and training for them, have validated the helpful, even necessary, confluence of a broader approach to therapeutic work with individuals, couples, families and groups

In this book, I hope to engage the reader through a set of arguments which focus on a few key terms and concepts. *Therapist* will be used throughout to identify a variety of professionals available to individuals and groups with the intent of ameliorating stress and conflict. Generically I shall refer to them as healers; the specificity of the reference will be grounded in the term therapist with the underlying assumption that their context is primarily secular.

Priest will connote a specifically spiritual context and worldview; a tradition of counseling within this framework may or may not include a formal religious context. Neither does the use of the term *priest* imply formal ordination even though there exists the presumption of a recognizable spiritual orientation and identity. *Spiritual realm* and w*orldview* are not exhaustively discussed but I will elaborate upon several fundamental principles regarding spirituality.

Two pivotal foundations for this thesis are: First, I will discuss the more generic definitions of spirituality in order to surround and support the assumptions I have made regarding the role I will eventually identify as *priestly*. Secondly, the discussion will present specific distinctions between religion as the more organized and structured entity in society and the religious aspirations of humankind that can be identified in descriptions of a person's capacity for *spirituality*. This discussion will also make it apparent that many see the very basis of our human longings as evidence of humankind's fundamental spiritual nature. The term *religious man* will be employed to reference this qualitative aspect of human experience.

To address the notion of *therapeutic*, I will draw from both general and specific understandings and definitions. It is important to note that some *healing* of life's pain and trauma happens naturally over time. My focus will be on those who intentionally seek help from an identified professional. Just deciding to make an appointment has decreased the level of stress in numerous cases. However, this thesis will look not only to those seeking help, but also to the spiritual resources available to both participants in the therapeutic relationship – seeker and healer; counselor and client; therapist and patient.

Chapter One elaborates on the roles of both therapist and priest as described in both classic and contemporary writings. Both of these established roles within a society or community will be approached within fundamental understandings surrounding *the professions*. Furthermore, I will describe these two *professions, therapist* and *priest*, as they relate to the notion of a call or vocation. Chapter One will conclude by citing arguments establishing both therapist and priest as belonging to ennobled professions.

Chapter Two defines and describes the role of therapist, and touches upon the concept of therapist as *healer*. The enlarged notion of therapist as healer elicits distinctions between therapist and priest. These distinctions also demonstrate a natural kinship between the vocations of priest and therapist. The priest as therapist, or vice versa, must also recognize the concept of *healer* which probably played a significant role in the priest's choosing a spiritual orientation.

Chapter Three continues the discussion of a person who both chooses and is called to communal responsibility for healing with the focus on a spiritual orientation. Critical to this discussion is the concept of mediator/atrix as it relates to the priestly dimension of healing. This section will present selected historical, philosophical and theological considerations pertaining to arguments linking therapists and priests as healers. Some of the similarities and distinctions between priestly and shamanic roles will be presented in view of their later relevance.

In **Chapter Four**, a modest discussion of the expansive and all too encompassing term *spiritual* is revisited. With a view to first touching upon the ubiquitous contemporary search for spirituality, it appears that the most fundamental, as well as basic etymological, considerations of the term *spiritual* leave open *de fine* the possibility, if not the probability, that the work of healing in the human community elicits something, or someone, larger than oneself.

As references to several authors from both the psychological and theological disciplines will demonstrate, that *larger good, higher power or non-material aspect* of the healing process has not only been understood to be a dynamic attending the one *seeking* help, but also a resource, even the source at some level, for those who consciously pursue and practice the healing professions. Understood and interpreted in light of these arguments, therefore, such professionals can be seen – and can choose to see themselves consciously and intentionally – as responding to a call to *be priestly, spiritually- grounded, healers.*

Available, therefore, to both those *seeking* growth, awakening, healing and human development, as well as to various practitioners of healing, this *greater good or higher power* can be a primary context and a consciously available collaborator in the healing process. I will also hasten to emphasize here what has been mentioned earlier and continues to operate as an important working assumption: Appropriate vocational preparation and theoretical foundations neither beg the question of things spiritual, nor do they in any way conflict with the therapeutic practice of any sort. A contrary position seems appropriate. Preparation for the practice of healing, through this lens, embraces the wisdom of science and the depths of fundamental understandings of both *spirituality* and *healing.*

Chapter Five will move the argument toward what can be seen as the spiritual dimensions of virtually any healing endeavor within either individual or communal contexts. Also presented is a discussion of *priestly* activity. Further role and identity distinctions within a discussion of *therapist as priest* will revisit the germane assumptions around spirituality and the notion of agency.

The efficacy of the healer, and therefore the healing taking place, has long been recognized as flowing from sound theoretical frameworks, careful training and preparation of the therapist-priest-healer. Obviously, the readiness of the one seeking help is also to be considered. When the *healer* is, at the same time, given to a belief, however secular it may need to be framed, that the dynamics in the healing process at least include, if not hinge upon, some other *spiritual* power, it can then be argued that those in the healing professions might well avail themselves of more than simply requisite knowledge, preparation and skills.

All features associated with the term therapist can indeed stand alone without a specifically, conscious, *religious* grounding. Purely scientific, empirical models of therapy continue to characterize the therapeutic relationship.

By elucidating the broader context of *spiritual,* and locating the work of healing within that framework, the role of healer has, of necessity and by definition, appropriate *priestly,* spiritual dimensions. *The therapist as priest* presents a role that incorporates traditional therapist characteristics yet also includes a spiritually based orientation, and, in a sense, a new treatment vocation. The *transpersonal* psychology orientation has adopted some dimensions of this position.

Bringing this work to its conclusion will be the task of **Chapter Six**. I propose that those who chose as their life's work the work of healing can also be aware of, and rely upon, the spiritual core of human life that *also chooses them* for their work as healers.

With concluding references to the work of Carl G. Jung, James Hillman, et. al., I will conclude that a therapeutic relationship, fully and rightly understood, and whether consciously referenced or not, rests fundamentally on spiritual foundations.

Chapter One
Professional Activity and Identity

Part I – The Professions

It has become rather commonplace to find the adjective *professional* describing almost any work-related activity or trade. If one needs proof of that statement, simply watch any highway long enough to observe any number of vehicles with the word *professional* painted in bold letters: *Professional Window Cleaning; Home Internet Professionals; Professional Drivers Wanted.* While I have no interest here in challenging the colloquial validity of persons choosing to think of themselves, or their work, as belonging to the professions, a more classic understanding of the professions is helpful in setting a context in which to address the roles of both therapist and priest.

In this chapter, I will set a context within which to begin a discussion of both therapeutic and priestly identities against a framework shaped by characteristics of professional identity and practice. It is my sense that the word *profession/al* has, over time and in some cultures like my own, come to connote that persons providing a professional service perform that service or trade full time. Hence, the inferences of a skill to which one's energies are devoted with single mindedness resulting in an outcome that is both reliable and carefully honed. Doing something with dedicated focus and resources suggest that one is *good at it, experienced.*

"Professional" vs
" Profession'

Furthermore, an implied connection seems present, whether intentionally placed or not, between such commonplace use of the word professional and some older connotations of the professions. As we shall see later, the older notions of *professional* stress the more selfless aspects of one's dedication not only to the professional endeavor, but also to the community. It also suggests that the professional's feelings of satisfaction outweigh monetary or material rewards. In this sense, the practice of one who is, and is recognized as, a *professional* in the community consciously ascribes to some level of altruistic goals in the carrying out of ones work.

I find current usage blurs the boundaries between skills well performed by reliable, courteous, full-time practitioners of various trades and services, and the more traditional professions as I would here typify them by referencing the medieval grouping of Theology, Medicine and Law.

The older medieval professions were divinity [theology], physic [medicine] and law. They were 'person professions' (Goode, 1969) centered on counselor-client relation. They did not produce goods for sale or works of art for enjoyment, but worked to heal, guide, or protect some person in a life crisis. [1]

Thus, professions in their more traditional sense center on persons, their field of expertise and a relationship between a counselor and client. The professional focus is understood to be a service involving a direct relationship between persons, not on the production of goods or on a service that does not directly affect the person served.

I stress again that this departure point in understanding, and applying, the notion of professional practice or behavior is disinterested in arguing the value or the propriety of assigning to the trades, or to those providing other services within the community, some of the same characteristics of competent or skilled service. I am emphasizing what several authors have consistently ascribed to early definitions of professional endeavors and the distinctions surrounding the nature of those professions: "...the value placed upon systematic knowledge and intellect: *knowing*. Second, the value placed upon technical skill and trained capacity, *doing*. And third, the value placed upon putting this conjoint knowledge and skill to work in the service of others, *helping*. [2]

Ethicists Ashley and O'Rourke offer a helpful listing of attributes that have traditionally attended the professions. The following description of professional behavior does not limit characteristics of good service to the professions alone. Yet it does set a useful standard against which to judge professional practice.

> Professional behavior may be defined in terms of four essential attributes: 1) a high degree of generalized and systematic knowledge; 2) primary orientation to the community interest rather than to individual self-interest; 3) a high degree of self control of behavior through codes of ethics internalized in the process of work socialization and through voluntary associations organized and operated by the work specialist themselves; and 4) a system of rewards [monetary and honorary] that is primarily a set of symbols of work achievement and thus ends in themselves, not means to some end of individual self-interest. [3]

While helpful in its outline of characteristic attributes, the definition fails to identify the expectancy of an outcome which, one hopes, is positive.

Yet critical to our use of the professions as a context within which to frame the roles of therapist and priest is this apparent emphasis in the older definitions of a profession, i.e., a primary orientation to the communal good over against self-interest. Identifying professional practice as distinct from other services and the trades hinges on this fundamental orientation to the community just as preparation and training for the various professions must, therefore, be informed and guided by it. This orientation, then, is a matter of both theory and practice. This communal orientation, we can assume, is a conscious, philosophical and deliberate underpinning that informs both preparation for professional practice as well as the standards used to certify, evaluate and monitor the activities of professional *praxis*.

Recall here that therapist is being used throughout this work to typify those who perform the task of healing from a largely psychosocial perspective. The therapist has an appropriate background in the social sciences and theoretical frameworks that enable him to engage in particular healing interventions.

Also, priest is being used throughout this work to typify those who perform the task of healing from a largely spiritual perspective. Priestly roles may connote both the general spiritual categories of human hungers and longing, as well as those attached to the various relgio-cultural perspectives of more organized faith groups. Another aspect of mediating healing to those served is the mutual recognition of a power greater than either the healer or the client in the relationship. Unlike magical paradigms of intervention, a greater presence available to both parties in the therapeutic relationship is simply acknowledged; it need not be named, and it is not sought after for the sake of control. Therapists and priests engaged in a counselor-client relationship more for the sake of the community than for their own self-interest are indeed people who rate high on the six operational attributes described by Moore and Rosenblum:

1. Professionals practice full time occupations.
2. They are committed to a calling, that is they treat their occupation as an enduring set of normative and behavioral expectations.
3. They are distinguished from the laity by various signs and symbols and are identified with their peers – often in formalized organizations.
4. They have esoteric but useful knowledge and skills through specialized *education* which is lengthy and difficult.
5. They are expected to have a service *orientation* so as to perceive the needs of a client relevant to their competency.
6. They have autonomy of judgment and authority restrained by responsibility in using their knowledge and skills. [4]

It is easy to understand, therefore, why authors like Ashley and O'Rourke, Barber, Moore & Rosenblum, Merton et. al. refer to such a system of rewards as "...primarily a set of symbols of work achievement and thus ends in themselves, not means to some end of individual self-interest [alone]." [5] Another author makes the same point by suggesting that

These four concerns – concerns for persons, trained skills, values and basic theory, and public responsibility – are the central themes of professional ideology always mentioned in the sociological literature on the professions and the professions' statement of purpose. [6]

By adding the teaching profession to those classic, medieval professions mentioned earlier – medicine, law and theology – we bring the primary foci and characteristics of the professions to four pivotal areas of community service. For not only do the endeavors of education, medicine, law and theology capture for us the most frequent professions mentioned in the literature concerning an early formulation of what it means to be a professional, these areas often intertwine in their very practice. This confluence of professional activity illustrate practically many of the points established thus far.

Medicine as both art and science clearly requires specialized knowledge, training and a commission, or licensure, to practice. As with the other professions mentioned, knowledge alone usually does not suffice once the goal of applying that knowledge to the persons served is neared. Our earlier mention of the fundamental aspect of a "counselor – client" relationship—so germane to professional practice – implicitly leads to the art of applying theoretical knowledge. In terms of medical practice, the 'counselor' becomes the examining physician in the individual case, and is assigned a position of responsibility for overseeing public health in the communal context. Likewise, the lawyer, teacher and spiritual advisor have obligations to the individual and the community.

In these professions, a general and specific knowledge base is applied to a given individual or communal presenting situation. The physician, in this example, is not only examining presenting symptomotology with a view to a differential diagnosis, he is also, no doubt, preparing to chart a course for care and counsel based on those clinical determinations. Knowledge, facts, findings become the basis for appropriate interventions. Those interventions may certainly include – especially in medical care and healing – pharmacology or surgery, but it is also true that physicians spend a good deal of office time simply listening and providing counsel on self-care, diet, exercise and the like. Even in medicine, so imbued with 'high tech' diagnostic and intervention tools, the physician is often more than doctor and the sick are more than patients. Though somewhat dated, one study showed that ...*fifty percent or more of patients seen by primary care physicians are not suffering from any physical dysfunction.* [7] A counselor–client relationship begins as soon as a patient steps into the office, or the community health department is put on alert.

Staying with this particular profession and example, it is also interesting to note the confluence and overlap of professional behavior and practice in the four classic professions we are using to typify and argue the thesis contained in the first chapter. Recall that it is here we are working to establish a framework and context within which to discuss and elaborate upon both therapist and priest as communal servants given a high degree of public, communal trust and responsibility. Here I continue to build the case that early notions surrounding who a professional is, and both how and why that public servant practices, is directly related to, and foundational for, the common ground uniting these two specific communal roles, i.e. *therapist and priest,* as servants to persons and to a greater good: Healing, health, wholeness; personal and communal development and well-being.

As a teacher works with the curious and those anxious to learn, so the physician and other healing professional do well to remember Hippocrates' early admonition to his followers on the island of Cos that the primary task of the physician is to engage the desire of the patient to be well. The professions, by definition, have in mind the good of those entrusted to their care.

Here I see a logical reason why human service and social science professionals evidence current interest in spirituality. Cross-disciplinary dialogue between spiritual counselors and therapists suggests the potential for a better outcome within each of the healing disciplines represented. In days past, a similar interest may have been present but not pursued. History shows that giving expression to it may have sent empiricists beyond the pale of serious scientific recognition.

In many cases, these stories and studies betraying the burgeoning interest in things spiritual signal both a popular hunger for, and a permission within the community of scientists and scholars to return to what Rudolf Otto called *that which is part of us, yet beyond us; the wholly other.* [8] This concept will be developed further in Chapter Four, yet it points once again to the important difference between a specific, formalized religious faith and the broader, spiritual, undogmatized human longings within us.

As a scientist, scholar and therapist, William Miller, for example, not only welcomes the change but also has labored professionally to assure that spirituality informs psychological theory and therapeutic activity. *What is new is the emergence of interaction between clinical science and spirituality, each informing the other. A taboo on incorporating spirituality in psychotherapy seems to be lifting, and nowhere has this taboo been stronger than in empirically oriented, scientist-practitioner circles.* [9]

In an article taken from a [US] weekly news magazine given almost entirely over to The *Search for the Sacred: America's Quest for Spiritual Meaning,* one contributing writer states that

> ...a funny thing has happened on the way to science's usurpation of the place of faith in the last years of the millennium. Among researchers as well as laypeople, discoveries in physics, biology and astronomy are inspiring a sense of cosmic piety, of serene holism and even a moral code. *I see a turnaround,* says Theologian Phillip Hefner, director of the Chicago Institute for Religion and Science, *in which many scientists are saying we can integrate science into an existing religion, a personal philosophy of life, or New Age beliefs.* [10]

On a the stage where religious ideation and spiritual exploration is not only receiving at least scientific curiosity, and in many cases serious attention that includes research and corroboration in distinct, though parallel, language, those who have given their professional lives to the study and interpretation of religious sentiment and spiritual hungers become credible colleagues and invaluable scholars alongside the scientific community. It is my view that this potent alliance is especially effective, and real, to the extent that both scientific empiricists and religious scholars are open to one another's findings and the underlying epistemology of each method.

In other words, biblical literalists -- or fundamentalists of any persuasion --setting out to prove what is tenaciously held *a priori* with no attention to the language of myth and symbol will add little to, and receive less from, a common effort to understand the spiritual hungers of humankind or the underlying truths contained within the meaning systems painted in religious stories, texts and language.

In contrast to such a religious reactionary posture, It is on this stage of mutual respect and wonder that scholars of religious history and meaning are called forth to assist professional colleagues in other disciplines who share their passion, intellect and responsibility for an individual's or a community's health, hungers, meaning systems and self-understandings in the context of culture and history. On this stage, history finds dialogue and debate rather than power positioning and turf protection which have traditionally drawn [often-violent] artificial lines between religion and science.

For our purposes here, it is especially on this stage, and in such a mutuality in the search for meaning and truth, that religious [*priests* et. al.] scholars [*educators*] stand alongside committed health [*healers/therapists*], legal and political [public servants] colleagues as true public servants and professionals sharing the kind of public trust assigned to their role within the community being served.

Part of the task in this thesis is to note the implicit connections between those who heal and serve the cause of human development from the more explicitly secular settings and disciplines [therapists] and those who serve as an individual's or a community's pastor, minister or spiritual guide [priest]. I have begun to set the stage for that thesis by arguing that in all the disciplines mentioned thus far, and in the practice of noble service to both individuals and to communities, those who are deemed professionals in the traditional sense are called to the kind of trust and public responsibility which will require of them more than a single, honed skill set akin to talented trade and craft persons.

Public servants who rise to such noble professions have been understood over time to be persons whose altruism may never be complete, nor without blemish and the earmarks of human failing and finitude, yet the very definition of a *professional* as we are using it treats such lofty goals of service to others as foundational to those positions. Consequently, when teachers, healers, clergy and politicians/leaders compromise their position and professional identity in activities of pure and obvious self-interest, disillusionment within the community about such persons and positions points to the often unspoken, but inherent, expectations surrounding their role.

I began this chapter by noting that some of the traditional distinctions between the *professions* and the *trades* are becoming progressively more blurred. Of particular interest in this thesis are those qualities of professional life and practice – including the explicit expectation in their formal training of the common good over self interest alone -- which certainly allow recompense for service rendered, but whose overarching purposes find fulfillment in a ...*system of rewards [monetary and honorary] that is primarily a set of symbols of work achievement and thus ends in themselves, not means to some end of individual self-interest.* [11]

As professionals who have been trained in their disciplines, and often mentored into their roles and responsibilities, therapists who heal from a more secular, scientific orientation and priests who do similar work from a more specific religious or spiritual perspective have been joined in this chapter at the levels of ... *the central themes of professional ideology always mentioned in the sociological literature on the professions and the professions' statement of purpose: These four concerns – concerns for persons, trained skills, values and basic theory, and public responsibility – are the central themes of professional ideology.* [12] Along with understanding that the task in this first chapter is to establish both therapist and priest as typifying two healing professions serving parallel, but distinct, roles on behalf of community members, I emphasize again that each of these role-identities is being used in a very generic way.

Keeping in mind that the task in the whole of my work is to establish the spiritual foundations of any therapeutic relationship, and that the title of the thesis betrays both it's focus and methodology -- Therapist *as* Priest – I will conclude this chapter with yet another important bridge which I see as inherent in the professions and arguably inherent in the work of all who could be typified as either therapist or priest: *Vocation.*

Part II – The Professional as one who is Called

Vocational Aspects of Professional Identity

Depth Psychologist and writer James Hillman is both a Jungian Scholar and Analyst and one of the few remaining students who knew Carl Gustav Jung personally and who was mentored by him. In his book, *The Myth of Analysis*, Hillman gives his entire first chapter over to rather candid, and sometimes very personal, reflections on how an *inner connection* begins to take shape between humans even before the actual physical encounter takes place. Almost paradoxically, Hillman ends this first chapter [entitled *Human Encounters and the Inner Connection*] by stating that *...the human encounter, as the first level of the counseling work, leads to the inner connection between the counselor and the counseled.* [13]

Yet he begins the same chapter with the clear conviction that to be an analyst, counselor, social worker means that one is waiting and wanting to heal [sometimes using the language of *trouble shoot* and *problem solving*] ... *even before the person comes in to take the waiting chair.* [14] He seems to suggest that there is already a foundational basis for the *connection* between seeker and healer based, at least in part, on the *need* of the counselor to be counselor, and the *call* emerging from that same need.

Stating that the meeting, or therapy session, begins not simply with the trained and organized intention of the professional helper but, in the case of analysis, the counselor's or analyst's response to a call to be healer initiates within him a desire to heal even before the contact begins. In analysis, Hillman argues, and, by extension, I would add in all professional practices where there is a *counselor-client relationship* of the kind we have discussed in this chapter, ... *we would say that the counter transference is there before the transference begins. My expectations are there with me as I wait for the knock on the door.* [15]

In fact, counter transference is there from the beginning since some unconscious call in me impels me to do this work... My needs are never absent. I could not do this work if I did not need to do this work. But my needs are not mine alone; at a deeper level they belong to, reflect, and speak from a situation which corresponds as well with the other's needs. Just as a person who comes to me needs me for help, I need him to express my ability to give help. The helper and the needy, the social worker and the social case, the lost and the found, always go together. [16]

Continuing this reflection with images that suggest a more than random, utilitarian pairing of gifts and needs among humans who encounter each other, Hillman moves into what is for him an important distinction between felt needs [which are often perceived as signs of weakness and dependence] and the notion of the call that brings one to the work he is compelled to do. While they may seem hardly to differ at first glance, needs taken seriously, and once they are redeemed from the simple negative perspective of weakness, can indeed betray a call – the root meaning of *vocation*.

But here it is necessary to note that needs and calls hardly differ. This tends to be experienced as coming more from without the personality, whereas needs seem "mine," coming from within. To deny a call is indeed dangerous, for it is a denial of one's essence which is transpersonal. But is not the denial of a need equally dangerous? Needs are not only personal. There is a level to them which is objective, so that, for instance, the need I feel to be with you is

13

not only my personal need but the objective requirement of the relationship we have, the voice which asks that it be kept alive. Need makes us human; if we did not need one another, if we could not meet and satisfy our own needs, there would be no human society. [17]

Whether cast in the language of need or of call, Hillman encourages us to be aware of, and honor, that we have human needs, and, furthermore, that those *needs* have a connection both to our call and to those we are called to be with. In the present context of Hillman's book and the work at hand in this chapter, the identification with the counselor – client connection is easily made.

So too, we have earlier demonstrated that one of the key elements in being a professional is precisely a person profession which is centered on a kind of counselor-client relationship that moves beyond what may be expected in a fair exchange of goods or services. Such an exchange, including the notion of a sales person interacting with a client, is applicable also in the trades. Yet in this kind of relationship where professionals engage in service to individuals or communities, we earlier noted Goode's assertion that professionals ...*did not produce goods for sale or works of art for enjoyment, but worked to heal, guide, or protect some person in a life crisis.* [18]

To be fair to even a brief treatment of James Hillman and the development of the counselor's call, he makes the equally important point that the *vocation* one senses, and then pursues through *what we know and have read, our gifts of intelligence and character – all we have gained through training and experience --* [19] can also get in the way of being a healthy counselor. He argues strongly, and pleads passionately, for any healer to be aware of the subtle distinctions between responding to a call to be someone, including a professional, and the unconscious urges to get one's human needs met while practicing that profession.

Hillman illustrates this at length in this first chapter by validating human needs as natural. He then argues that such needs play a real role in helping a person, in this case a counselor or analyst, discover what path to follow in his or her life's work. Furthermore, the need to train, prepare for and become the professional counselor that suits his needs will be met in the human encounters where he will engage with those who have need of that service. More caveats follow, however, for the well-intentioned, but all too ego-driven, consciousness of the therapist.

Just as any counselor can turn the consulting session into fruitful, effective clinical hour for the healer, the efficacy of the therapeutic encounter will not only be questionable, but it is destined to be lost entirely in a sea of subjectivity if the professional healer casts the seeker into the problem the counselor is most ready, able and needing to solve.

What might this mean, and how does the healer's need to be effective find its way into our discussion of the vocational dimensions of those who would be professionals?

Hillman is supporting the notion of call, or vocation, even as he cautions his readers against what he calls the evils of *curiosity*. In an admonition well known to those who have had any training in the work of therapy, Hillman addresses what is commonly understood to be pivotal for those practicing the healing arts and sciences: self-awareness.

In saying that ...*psychology cannot avoid beginning with the psychologist,* [20] Hillman is no doubt referring to the standard practice in analytical [depth] psychology of the analyst being trained coterminous with extensive self-analysis, and then continuing his own analysis while caring for others. Yet I know of no training program for therapists or spiritual directors of any stripe which does not require the student to be in therapy/direction, or, when finally practicing, being under clinical/spiritual *supervision* [at minimum during an initial training or certification period] – or both. While the rationale in any of the therapeutic disciplines may be obvious, the point to be made about avoiding one's own, unbridled, unconscious needs as a healer makes such a requirement noteworthy as we discuss the *professional practice* of therapy under the aegis of *vocation.*

From the Jungian perspective, and in the words of Hillman, working consistently at one's own self-awareness, in whatever subset of the counseling disciplines, is the primary way to avoid turning the seeker into one who will meet both the need and the call of the professional healer regardless of the felt needs of the one who knocks on the door. Within the larger context of the work seen as vocation, such a requirement may also provide assurance that the professional at best continues to feel called and practices competently; and at worst avoids harm by remaining in a vocation in which he no longer finds meaningful, professional vitality.

> A counselor may need to instruct and educate, to teach what he knows, because it fulfills an essential part of himself. It evokes his specific *call* [emphasis mine] to action. Yet he can hardly demand that each person coming to him each visit come only for instruction. His need to teach may have to find other fulfillment, else it may become an unconscious demand on each person who comes to him. If I admit my need for analytical work, I may demand less from those who come. Because demands build up when needs are not admitted, acknowledgment of my needs subjectively, as a fact of my humanity, my dependent creatureliness, will help to prevent

those same needs from degenerating into demands for actual fulfillment upon the objective world. Demands ask for fulfillment, needs only require expression. [21]

Self-awareness, which has already been identified as a critical part of rendering appropriate service to the client based on the client's needs and best interest, is demanded of the counselor-in-training, as well as the professional in practice, to both prepare that person for the right practice of the profession, and to ensure that self-interest, or the therapist's needs, have minimal power in the consulting room.

Self-awareness as it is required of the *therapist-healer* while performing ones professional role is also mirrored in many of the application processes requisite for professional training. Witness the application packets provided by schools which prepare attorneys, physicians, clergy and counselors. Prior academic achievements and transcripts alone represent only part of required documentation. Prospective students are traditionally asked for an autobiographic self-reflection statement inclusive of a statement describing ones life goals, or reasons for making application. Such self-assessment is often required prior, or in addition to, the program's standard aptitude test requirements. These suggest that while it may be helpful to know why a person wants to learn trade skills such as auto mechanics or dental hygiene techniques, some knowledge of, and dedication to, the more altruistic goals of a profession are inherently part of the discernment process for both applicant and mentor-instructors. A successful outcome for the student is not the sole consideration here, just as intellectual capacity and ability to acquire, and eventually perform, required tasks or skills will not, in and of themselves, fulfill the requirements of professional practice as we have outlined them above. Ascendancy to positions of public trust and responsibility involve a *counselor-client relationship.* It is primarily in that relationship, and the ability of the professional to navigate it within the framework of the particular professional paradigm, that the contribution to individuals, communities and a greater good is served – often with a minimum of monitoring and a maximum of trust. Being called to such service is a process which is best discerned by both a willing servant as well as those representing the greater good to be served.

Commenting on the gradual depersonalization of the professions, Ashley and O'Rourke wonder aloud

> Will professionals become technocrats whose technological mastery must extend itself to behavior control? Or will they become the persons to help others to transcend the depersonalization of technological systems in order to free them from what Alain Touraine calls 'dependent participation.' If professionals choose the latter alternative, then the professions must again be personalized... [professionals themselves have been depersonalized by loss of a clear identity]...and contributing to this confusion of identity today is the tension within the professions between the goals of research and the goals of practice ... many areas of professional practice may soon be handed over to computers. How then can a professional make that kind of commitment always regarded as a mark of the profession if it is not clear to what he or she is professed? [22]

Chapter One Notes

1 Ashley, Benedict M. & O'Rourke, Kevin D.: *Health Care Ethics* [1982] The Catholic Health Association of the United States, St. Louis, MO., pg. 79
2 ibid., pg. 81
3 ibid.
4 ibid. pg. 82
5 ibid.
6 ibid., pg. 81
7 ibid., pg. 100
8 Otto, Rudolf: *The Idea of the Holy* [1967] Oxford University Press, London pg. 25
9 Miller, William R. [ed.]: *Integrating Spirituality Into Treatment* [1999] American Psychological Association, Washington DC, pg. xiii
10 *Newsweek* Magazine, November 28, 1994, New York, NY; Special Edition: *The Search for the Sacred, America's Quest for Spiritual Meaning* Pg. 56
11 Ashley and O'Rourke, op. cit., pg. 81
12 ibid. pg. 81
13 Hillman, James: *Insearch* [1967] Spring Publications, Dallas, Texas, pg. 39
14 ibid., pg. 16
15 ibid., pg. 17
16 ibid.
17 ibid.
18 Ashley and O'Rourke, pg. 79
19 ibid. pg. 16
20 Hillman, James: *Insearch* [1967] Spring Publications, Dallas, Texas, pg. 16
21 ibid., pg. 18
22 Ashley and O'Rourke, Op. Cit. pg. 80

Chapter Two
Therapist as Healer

Part I – The Context

This thesis began with a personal reflection in the preface. I did this, in part, not only to establish something of a particular, personal backdrop for my passionate interest in the spiritual dimensions of healing, and those of a therapeutic relationship, but also to trace a chronology of experience which led me to conclusions I felt I could defend in an academic thesis. Another way to express this is to say that what I learned in the study of theology and spirituality, that what I experienced in the practice of ministry and what I saw coming to the fore in both scholarly and news magazine journals was precisely that which I was taught and experienced in the work of healing from a spiritual perspective during ministry years.

Utilizing scientific, empirically based formulations of human growth, development, change and illness alongside a philosophical anthropology distinguished by its openness to a spiritual reality beyond oneself has the best chance of appropriating all that is real in the work of healing -- of helping to make whole. By example, those of us who entered our post-graduate theological training -- four rather intense years in my tradition – in the late 1960's found that curricula previously focused almost solely on theological and spiritual disciplines now included a scattering of courses designed to bridge theology and psychology under the aegis of *pastoral counseling and psychology*. In my major seminary experience [1968 –

1972], pastoral *psychology* courses were taught by professionals degreed in the social sciences and brought into the heretofore insular walls of theologically focused training. While this is more than commonplace today, such transitions in theological curricula suggested both the practical wisdom of their inclusion, as well as the prior long years of professional dialogue among the disciplines in question.

I use an experiential reference in this chapter for the sake of pointing to the other side of the equation as well: We ought not miss the simple truth that degreed professionals, including practicing, doctoral level therapists, were willing and capable of crafting and teaching pastoral psychology out of 1) their interest in the convergence of these two disciplines; 2) the literature and research around such convergences already available; and 3) the hard fought conviction within the walls of seminaries like my own that graduate programs preparing priests should bridge spiritual and psychological development.

Since our focus in this chapter is on the therapist as healer, the point to be made in this example comes more from the fact that secular therapists and academicians given to the social sciences had both the resources available to them and the interest in bridging the connections from their own study and professional disciplines to those studying, and preparing to *professionally practice*, if you will, theology and spirituality. Again, it is worth noting that from our contemporary vantage point such a phenomenon, and such collaboration, seems unremarkable. I use the term common sense above in order to highlight the *permission*, as well as the deemed necessity [by the late 1960's] of demonstrating and applying the dialogue taking place within and between theology and psychology. Course offerings in *pastoral counseling and psychology*, while now a standard requisite for ministry professionals, were the early, and sometimes first, results of a cross disciplinary dialogue and its academic expression [*praxis*] within the walls of a previously carefully monitored, and sometimes suspicious, Roman Catholic seminary.

As we have mentioned several times, both psychological and spiritual care have for their focus *individuals* and *communities* seeking help. We, as pastoral professionals, would be sent to serve both. It made eminent sense to enter the dialogue and embrace both theoretical and practical insights for the sake of our own preparation as leaders and caregivers with the focus kept on those we would be sent to serve. That, indeed, is yet another – however simple – way of framing some of the material we have treated in this paper regarding the vocational focus of any professional.

I return now to the identity of the therapist, and to some of the history that informs both the natural connection to scientific, secular interest in things spiritual and to the common ground, rooted in the notion of a professional calling, which such healers have shared with more specifically spiritual practitioners of healing. However, the emphasis in this chapter will be more on the identity and work of those I have gathered into secular, scientifically based, healers. The foundational connection between therapist and priest in this, and the following chapter, will be primarily that of a professional called to a kind of service wherein significant training, specialized knowledge and skill, self-supervision, internal mechanisms of organizational standards and monitoring, rewards as a set of symbols and the counselor-client relationship as sacred are pivotal. It will be the work of the final chapter and summary, as indicated in the introduction, to address the spiritual foundations of a therapeutic relationship, and thus argue conclusively that the therapist has a priestly function.

Keeping in mind this image of a time when I and many others experienced in practical ways how and why these *secular* social scientists were called upon to inform our spiritual development and academic preparation, let me turn to this chapter's focus: The Therapist as Healer.

Part II – A Brief Look at Divergence and Departure: Medicine and Magic

The fertile land between the Tigris and Euphrates rivers is thought to be the cradle of medicine. Simple illnesses were diagnosed and treated by family members; more serious illness required shamanic or religious intervention –or both. More will be said about these distinctions in the chapter on Spirituality.

Depending on the time in history and the type of society, serious illness that did not respond to whatever *ordinary* treatment regimes perceived by a community as efficacious, early diagnostic categories were often discussed and available treatments were applied. Possible causes for grave illness included harm done by another person; a demon introduced as a foreign body; a punishment from a deity for sin; or full possession of the body by a demon. There is evidence to suggest that the diagnostic agent's fees were determined in some cultures by the accuracy of the prognosis.

Babylonian priest-physicians searched for omens – the stars, a flickering candle, a drop of oil – to prognosticate the fate of their patients. If the person's fate were death, the priest-physician would not treat the patient for fear of interfering with destiny. Incantations were more frequently used in treatment than were herbs, drugs or physics.

Atkinson asserts that Egypt is the birthplace of medical science, yet notes that until a century and a half ago it was a land clothed in mystery. Myths about its medical contributions prevailed until newly found papyri steadily replaced them with greater historical detail.

From the first dynasty onward, Egypt had a system of medicine more traditional than the world was again to see for over three thousand years. Egyptian physicians famous as teachers visited and taught in

Arabia, Persia and Greece. Hippocrates, grandfather of the physician by that name, was the pupil of an Egyptian. Medical knowledge in Greece, fused with Egyptian teaching, was handed down from father to son as a family heritage. In this way, Egyptian medicine became the groundwork for Greek medicine as given to us by Hippocrates. [23]

Though we now know that many physicians contributed to the *science* of medicine before he lived, Hippocrates has for centuries been called the *Father of Medicine*. Even if others in history have more accurately demonstrated a careful trial and error approach to the art of healing, his departure from magical incantations and the suggestion that all sickness has a natural cause makes him an appropriate reference point in medical history.

For the early Greeks, there were two gods of healing. IMOUTHES, himself a physician, was given post-mortem divine status and associated with ASKLEPIOS. The Asklepiads believed in faith healing through placebos and miraculous temple cures. The sick were actually boarded in the temple with hope for a miraculous cure.

Sleeping in the temple seemed to cause a state of rest reminiscent of a hypnotic state. During such sleep, suggestions were often made in the hope that the deeper spirit of the sick, as well as the gods, would listen and respond. In some areas during this fourth century B.C. period of Greece, the sick were brought to public places in order that passers-by might recommend the treatments that had aided them.

Hippocrates formed a school for the healing arts and his early followers organized into a guild with ASKLEPIOS as its patron. Together they began what we might think of as empirical medicine: The guild began to repeat successful treatments without any attempt at defining illness or discovering why certain therapeutics worked. By observing and recording therapeutic effects, these early physicians began the process of distinguishing medical healing from priestly divinations.

The corpus of work surviving these Hippocratic guilds is small. Yet it does appear that any tension between the early Greek medicine of this period and the parallel, religious interventions of temple authorities might mimic the perennial tension between medicine and magic, science and faith. At least on Hippocrates' island of Cos, and in the shadow of ASKLEPIOS' temples, priests were retained as healers, but in ways more familiar to our contemporary experience.

> It is clear that all physicians of the time had the same ideas in common, that physical conditions to a marked degree would respond to mental states. The function of the priest-healer then was to direct the patients' mind into wholesome channels. Next to this came the art of dietetics in treating the sick. All Greek schools of medicine taught the sick to select their food well, to eat less and thus to live longer. Third in the list of help to the sick was that of drugs. There were few of these, chief among them being purgatives, and these were only seldom administered. But the patient was urged to eat deliberately, to chew his food well, and seek repose after meals. [24]

How Hippocrates came to free his mind of magic is not known. Neither is it known how he managed to gain such vast knowledge of diagnoses and treatment. Whatever the route, his treatise on the *Sacred Disease* – an illness now known to us as epilepsy – was a significant manifestation of his distaste for the theory that disease resulted from a visitation of the gods. *Here he used the term only to identify it [Sacred Disease], and states that the 'falling sickness' was not, in fact, any more sacred than other diseases which visited upon mankind, but that it had a natural cause which was not understood.* [25]

Magic – defined as *any attempt to manipulate and control destiny by practices and substances thought to contain inherent supernatural power* [26] has found its way into medicine and religion in various ways and at several points in history. While it is possible for religion and medicine to coexist and even inform one another, *magic, by its very nature impinges upon human concerns which properly belong to medicine, thus conflicting with any medical system that is not magico-religious.*[27] Amundsen and Gerngren further point out that *magic has retained its basic characteristics over the centuries, while both religion and medical systems have changed a great deal.* [28]

Whether early departures from medicine of magico-religious thinking began decidedly in Greek practice, solidified with the rise of the European University systems or simply faded away except in area where cultures remained steeped in animism, healing of the mind and body eventually looked to natural causes and remedies. This brief section, by it's location in Chapter Two, not only informs this chapter's material concerning the therapist as healer, but provides a starting point for references in Chapters Three and Four around distinctions between priest as healer [III] and spirituality [IV] .

Part III – The Medical Model as Informing Healers' Identity and Methods

Having briefly touched on early departures from magical world views as causative, and therefore, curative of disease [as well as *dis-ease*], it is important to at least touch upon the rise and influence upon healing modalities of a decidedly secular, medical model. This model highlighted the physical aspects of symptoms and diagnosis, as well as the choice of treatment options. This form of medicine's diagnostic and treatment approach evolved slowly and in different expressions across time and geography; it took firm root with the rise in Europe of the university system.

Although history suggests a tenacious connection between many forms of medicine and spirituality, empirical science took hold in ways that often left behind a general sense that

> Spiritual well-being is an important and too often overlooked dimension of health. Much is already known. Spiritual and religious involvement is not only common but is often important in clients' lives and has been generally linked to positive health outcomes. A client's spiritual perspectives may be relevant in understanding his or her problems and useful in the process of treatment. Although seldom taught in the training of health professionals, there is a large literature on the assessment of spirituality and religiousness. Incorporating spiritual perspectives in secular treatment has been found to improve outcomes for religiously oriented clients. Spiritually rooted interventions and collaboration with spiritual professionals may also enhance a successful treatment. [29]

The truth remains that the medical model not only rose to a place of prominence in treatment modalities, in many educational and professional training programs it was the model that informed – implicitly or explicitly – the practice of healing. As Dr. Miller comments in his *Integrating Spirituality Into Treatment*:

As scientific methodology increasingly came to guide medical treatment, the health professions became differentiated, first as secular, then as a proliferating array of subspecialties. A medical-technological model emerged as the dominant paradigm in medicine as well as well as psychology and other health professions that emulated it. Implicit assumptions of this view are that a) differential diagnosis [i.e., the identification of the disease or disorder] is the crucial first step; b) each disease has a definable specific cause; c) there is an identifiable best treatment to eradicate the cause; and d) technological specialization is optimal in the treatment of the disease. This model has been effective in treating certain [e.g., infectious] diseases, although even there it may fail by overlooking social, psychological, environmental, and behavioral dimensions of illness. [30]

This remarkable work whose very publication by the American Psychological Association [1999] signals both the permission the social sciences are embracing in approaching the subject, as well as the felt need among psychologists, psychiatrists, social workers et. al. for the material presented, captures succinctly a current trend back to spirituality as it informs therapeutic modalities. Contributors Miller and Thoresen are among many health professionals urging mutual collaboration between professionals in the Philosophical, Theological and Spiritual traditions and those whose life has been given to the scientific study of human behavior. In doing so, they not only touch upon a lack of preparation around spiritual dimensions of health in most clinical training models, but they also suggest a basic remedy toward a better outcome. Their writing lends credence to what ethicists Ashley and O'Rourke site as a common etiology of both *sacred and profane* concern for health and wholeness; indeed, the common roots of healing. Commenting that the *...two aspects of medical education [which] have always coexisted and still do, i.e., orthodox scientific medicine and a vast field of heretical medicine ...ranging from naturopathy, faith healing, homeopathy, and chiropractic to osteopathy, acupuncture, and 'holistic' medicine... not to mention countless forms of pure quackery* [31] ... the authors trace both recent, scientific forms of healing and more explicitly spiritual approaches to both a common source and a fundamental human longing.

> This duality, upon closer examination, reflects the mind-body or psychosomatic duality of the human being who is sick. In early times, the learned professions all originated from the one rather confused profession of priest [or perhaps priest-king]. Priests were looked upon as custodians of sacred wisdom and power over the forces of nature, a gift from the gods who alone possessed cosmic secrets... [32]

Yet we are using the term therapist to refer to the secular, psychosocial modalities of healing. While I have established a common footing for both therapists understood in that light, and priests as more spiritually based healers, through a discussion of common attributes attending the professions [Chapter One], Ashley and O'Rourke's further insights are pertinent. As ethicists and historians, they help us understand the common, priestly character and origin of the healing professions. At the same time, they enable our focus – especially in this chapter – on more recent, secular contexts [professions] whose historical development, scientific framework and distrust of subjective, spiritual categories of experience eventually led to what we typify as pivotal in the medical model of healing. In *Health Care Ethics* they write,

> In strong contrast to the psychotherapeutic models,... the patient enters both models in much the same kind of setting – a private office, clinic or hospital. In the medial model, the professional goal is to treat a physical illness so as to restore normal physical functioning to the degree possible. The physician first seeks to diagnose the disease, then prescribe a course of treatment (in which the physician is assisted by nurses and others) through medicine, surgery, nursing or change of regime. The physician must also make a prognosis and, if possible, offer the patient hope. The patient, on the other hand, is relieved from blame for his or her condition and from ordinary responsibilities to work and family, but is expected to be cooperative with the professional staff. ... In this model, the patient is not expected to be as active as in the psychotherapeutic model except in the rehabilitative stages of treatment...[33]

Unquestionably engaged in a counselor-client context, the physician in this model attends to, and focuses on, the presenting physical illness toward the *restoration of normal physical functioning to the degree possible*. The anecdotal way of describing this focus comes to mind when I remember how many time during my ten years as hospital chaplain I heard a staff colleague say to me, and sometimes literally, *the gallbladder in room 203 asked to see you.* The truth is that the requesting patient had had her gallbladder surgically removed, and so another staff member, equally immersed in a subtle, but strongly impersonal, medical framework may have said *the cholecystectomy* had asked for a visit! Either way, there was little question about what brought the patient into care, what diagnosis followed and what the latest medical treatment indicated for care and cure.

Lest this remembered characterization of an environment saturated with skillful medical interventions and knowledgeable, professional healers seem unfairly reductionistic to a lack of either genuine care or professionalism as we have earlier described it, we note again the goals implicit in the medical model support such a technological, surgical intervention: Differential diagnosis; treatment options and planning; appropriate and scientifically established interventions.

Yet even in this model, so familiar and effective in settings where physical illness is likely to respond to known treatments, the priestly role of the physician continues to be discussed in medical history and journals even though a medical student may never be required to consider it in any formalized training component or hear it named explicitly in residency training. Nonetheless, early origins of healing and therapy seem to haunt even the halls of science if not the minds and hearts of those who heal.

> ...the physician to this day retains something of a priestly ministry in the service of the healing forces of nature. Something similar is true of every profession, because all professions deal with the sacred dignity of the human person and rest on the sacred covenant of trust between client and professional. [34]

Ethicists and scholars of medical history Ashley and O'Rourke are Dominican priests. We are not surprised, then, by their sensitivity and attention to the *spiritual*, more subjective aspects of healers' ministrations even within this scientific model. Yet as ethicists, they ground such convictions not on the personal faith, attitude or kindness of medical caregivers as much as they do upon a foundational element belonging to the *professions* and to which we have referred earlier: The counselor-client relationship.

As noted in Chapter One, this relationship is both a fundamental aspect of the professions which distinguishes them from those where goods are sold and services are rendered. The very nature of the professional relationship transcends the two persons [or groups] consciously entering into it by reason of the implicit responsibilities of the *counselor* and the explicit expectations belonging to the *professions* as described in Chapter One. Along with communal expectations for lofty goals and trusted, selfless service, persons feeling a *call* to such positions of service, and who are willing to undergo often-rigorous programs of preparation and training, freely and consciously accept positions of trust, responsibility and the artful application of their knowledge in ways that respect the dignity and rights of their clients. Precisely because of the implicit expectations of the professions on the part of those served, and in order to make more explicit the nature of the relationship, professionals often transition to communal positions of trust and responsibility by way of symbols that go beyond the typical rites of transition or graduation.

Oaths of service and responsibility take different forms: Symbols of service might be transferred; Investiture often takes place; licenses to practice and apply their knowledge follow upon academic degrees signifying the attainment of academic standards and theoretical competencies. It is from the level of knowledge and skill combined with a professional mantle of responsibility and willingness to uphold professional goals and standards that the notion of a communal contract edges closer to an older notion of covenant. While it easy to see that a professional counselor-client relationship is of such import that it lends itself to both implicit and explicit contractual and mutually acknowledged expectations about the kind, and the nature of, the services to be rendered to persons and to communities, the foundational trust between both parties seems to call forth earlier, commonly held origins of professional identity and activity. Drawing upon notions captured more by theological than legal inference, some authors have placed professional relationships in the context and nuance of covenant.

Once again using the physician as an example of secular healers typifying those working from a more empirically objective, scientific professional posture, Ashley and O'Rourke argue that ...*fundamental to [this] contract is the physician's concern for the patient's well-being.* Furthermore, ...Trust *will never exist if the patient believes that the physician is concerned only about the fee or acting out of mere routine like a machine or bureaucratic functionary.* With language connecting us to lofty, professional goals, individual and communal responsibilities, and aspirations beyond their own material success, the authors remind medical professionals that they [physician-healers] *must communicate interest in the patient as person, not as a kidney or heart, and a willingness to do for the patient whatever is professionally possible, not limited by mere self-interested motives.* ... [35]

For this reason, Paul Ramsey has

...rightly emphasized that the professional contract is something more than a contract; it is a 'covenant' in the theological sense. ... in that the professional undertakes to help the client not because the client is ethically worthy of help, nor even because he is able to pay for the service, but primarily because of the human need and the essential human rights based on need rather than merit. ... Health care professionals have the fundamental responsibility, within their specialties, to be expert in both the science and the art of health care, up-to-date in knowledge, experienced, of good judgment and skilled in procedures. Personal warmth does not substitute for [medical] expertise. Reciprocally, however, it may be said that this knowledge and skill cannot be put to their best use if the other humanistic elements are not also present. [36]

Part IV – Extending the Medical Model: Healing and Therapy

I have already cited attributes of the professional character as well as a foundational, common link underlying professional practice: a position of trust and communal responsibilities which place service over self-interest. I have argued that this professional identity serves also to establish a foundation for both therapist and priest as healers. So, too, we saw in the previous sections of this chapter, and by extension of the physician as belonging more to the secular, scientific healing professions, that the priestly quality of their craft comes not only from the nature of the professional - client relationship, but from the dignity of the human person[s] served. Chapter One addressed the counselor-client relationship and identified that the role of counselor applies to the professional dimension of secular healers in ways that go beyond what is typically thought of as counseling *per se*. We noted earlier that ministers, educators, attorneys-at-law and healers of the body all have a counseling role; all of them, too, relate to individuals and communities in that counseling, advocacy, advisory and consultative capacities.

In this chapter, we are treating the therapist as a secular-based healer; that is, one whose professional commitment, role and relationship with individuals and communities betray conscious and discernable attributes of professional behavior. The professional role of counseling when applied to, and practiced by, a therapist, takes on a broad range of emphasizes, foci, foundational theories and therapeutic modalities which depend on the school of thought giving birth to the particular goal and purpose seen to be the task of the therapeutic intervention.

The psychoanalytic school will differ in theory and practice from the depth psychological perspective. Some practitioners will employ the teachings of Erik Erickson, while others will favor Milton Ericson. A gestalt approach may inform many approaches, while a rehabilitation model may focus narrowly, and with no apology, on the psycho-educational approach to therapy and concern itself largely with cognitive and behavioral change. The point to be made is that style of treatment, use of pharmaceuticals, length of treatment and dynamics of setting, e.g., family systems work over against individual therapy, group process as compared to reliance on psychoactive drugs with a minimum of monitoring etc., differ widely based on a number of variables in both the presenting problem and the orientation, skills and training of the treatment professional.

Yet any theoretical framework, any resulting treatment approach, must start somewhere. To be a therapist of any persuasion, a professional counselor belonging to any school, or, indeed, even the choice and ability to apply an eclectic, multi-dimensional approach to psychological health, begins in the notion of who and what a therapist *is* beyond his professional identity and areas of competence. It is difficult to frame the *is-ness*, or essence, of the therapist without some reference to what he *does* within the professional context. As that context already includes some form of counselor-client relationship, both the need of the client approaching and the vocational need [cf. discussion of Hillman, Chapter One] of the therapist-healer must include the question of who the professional therapist is.

In a book entitled *Models of Madness, Models of Medicine,* authors Miriam Siegler and Humphrey Osmond [1974] identified eight potential models of therapeutic relations. While it is true that this particular work springs from the experience of two authors whose professional training and practice fall decidedly within the medical model of healing, their work and interest in various forms of counselor-client relationships take a wider view and include other healing professionals. While they in fact name and describe eight models of possible therapeutic styles, relationships and the implicit dynamics of each – as well as influences and styles flowing between those named – it is the psychoanalytic approach, together with other authors' commentary on it, which will be most helpful in the therapist's role as healer and the foundational way that his identity is constellated. Still, in the counselor-client relationship one must appreciate the needs of both the client [seeker] and the therapist [healer] in the relationship.

As summarized by Ashley and O'Rourke, the psychoanalytic model is that framework and process *...whereby the therapist assists the patient to come to a greater self-knowledge, even of unconscious motivation, and to develop a more effective way of living.* [37] Precisely how, why and over what length of time that happens, if indeed it does, is obviously much more complex, and certainly varied, in theoretical and stylistic approaches within a broad, even if specific, school of thought, and, finally, shaped by both the presenting problem [client/patient] as well as particular professional practitioner. I find, however, that these authors, together with the Ashley/O'Rourke commentary, present a basic, broad-based view regarding who the therapist as healer *is*:

> ...the client comes to the therapist because of painful anxieties that make normal life difficult or impossible, with the goal of trying to resolve emotional conflicts whose unconscious origin is unknown to the client. The therapist's responsibility is ... to help the client come to an understanding of the causes of his or her problems and to cope with them more effectively. To achieve this, the therapist must gradually win the client's trust and help the client, gradually, to interpret the symbolism of the symptoms. The therapist must grant the client the right to have his or her

behavior interpreted rather than judged morally and to have the client's sufferings counted worthy of sympathy ... to discover their underlying meaning, and thus come to a deep and realistic self-understanding. Finally, the therapist must help the client discover new skills in coping with the problems of life and terminate dependence on the therapist. To do this, the therapist must personally arrive at self-understanding through the same process.

The client must come to trust the therapist, speaking more and more freely, cooperating by undertaking the task of working through the symptoms, rejecting escape from the process ... The client's will to get well and become independent of the therapist must also be reinforced. This process depends on an intense one-to-one relation in which the patient withdraws from the familial and social situation in which he has become ill. [38]

The above is more a description of the therapist-healer than it is a definition. To *define* is to literally *set limits* [lat. *de-fine*], or discover where the territory contained in the definition starts and ends. Yet, as we describe this particular orientation of healer, and who that healer is from a scientifically informed, secular perspective, we immediately see that at least eight models of healers emerge, and each of the eight may well have multiple situational and theoretical emphases. In choosing the above narrative-description seated within a particular psychoanalytic model, my belief that one cannot speak of the *is-ness* of the therapist without detailed discussion of both the client-patient *seeker* and the counselor-client relationship is concretely represented. The descriptive narrative above, while one of perhaps hundreds, does not attempt to discus the therapist's role without some mention of basic, fundamental requisites flowing from awareness of pain to the desire for health and how those two elements are engaged, then deepened, in the healing process.

Part V – Concluding Remarks – The Therapist

Treating who the therapist *is* and how any particular *therapeutic* modality operates as applied to, and informs, the secular, scientific identity of *healer* has been framed within the foundational context of the professions. Chapter One elucidates those starting points and took care to demonstrate how both *therapist* and *priest* belong to the professions by the several theoretical and practical attributes attending professional identity, preparation, self-awareness and practice. In Part Two of that same chapter, I turned to Jungian scholar and depth psychologist [*analyst*] James Hillman as I began some discussion of call, or vocation, as it pertains to the work of therapy and the dynamics of the therapeutic encounter. This section of this chapter is now the appropriate time and place to discuss more explicitly my choice of post-Freudian psychologies generally, and the analytical emphases in particular.

I earlier employed the professional role of physician-healer in order to address medicine's departure from magic [in the medical model] as well as to locate even this decidedly scientific approach to healing in a more subjective, priestly, tradition. Turning now to the more narrow focus of psychological healing, I find it useful to frame such a healer's identity against a modern, albeit relatively short, period of psychological thinking which entered with Freud. Beginning there also allows me to depart from that place. The wider purview of thinkers who moved on from Freudian thought provides a context for my argument as I end this chapter on the *therapist as healer.*

In drawing attention to some of the major departing points of at least two schools influenced by Freud -- Adlerian and Jungian -- I find that a larger post-Freudian view returned to healing from the psychological perspective just as balance returns to medicine when all aspects of the professional *counselor-client relationship* mark legitimate, sound medical practice. While the priestly, spiritual character of the therapist is indeed a central theme in these pages, the identity of the therapist cannot be discussed without mention of a broader view of how that professional works with a client; his own perspective, or self-identity, as healer or therapist at levels that exist and operate beyond orientation or a particular psychological framework. Here, therefore, I too need to move beyond Freud's contribution if only to set that larger context and welcome what scientists, whether medical or social, have too often collapsed into the subjective.

Raymond Corsini's *Current Psychotherapies* [second edition] lists thirteen schools of thought gathered under the book's title. To be sure, one can find variations on each of those treated in his compendium: Psychoanalysis; Adlerian and Analytical Psychotherapy; Person-Centered and Rational-Emotive Therapy; Behavioral Psychotherapy; Gestalt and Reality Therapy; Experiential Psychotherapy; Transactional Analysis; Psychodrama; Family Therapy; Human Potential. [39]

Given the edition's [second, revised] publication date of 1979, there is little doubt that subsets attached to any of the broader schools may already have argued for separate titles and status. Indeed, today's therapy conferences and journals are replete with abbreviations announcing both new emphases and new forms of treatment. Over the years, segmented, smaller schools which seem to nuance larger frameworks often coalesce into broader, thematic approaches to theory and practice [in psychology]. Many of these find genuine interest within the field, if not significant support. The Transpersonal Psychology movement, for example, seems less associated today with a kind of Californian propensity for the unorthodox, and more centrist in returning to the ancient roots of psychology found in metaphysics.

Corsini's listing of the 'Current Psychotherapies,' however, serves two basic, simple functions in approaching a description of the therapist and the therapist's work of healing.

First, it obviates the multiplicity of theoretical frameworks that have been formulated, researched and put forward in academic and professional training. Second, it locates the historical framework for this chapter's reference to the broad sweep of psychology and therapy within the relatively short period of time that begins with the work of Freud and the Psychoanalytic school. That is not to say, however, that either this final section of Chapter Two, or the thesis itself, adopts the view that either psychology or therapy is limited in definition, or origins, to this identifiable period. In fact, many volumes representing many schools of therapeutic thought contain this sort of language and historical notation by way of preface or introduction:

> Attempts to forge a systematic and inclusive understanding of human behavior by no means originated with contemporary Western psychology. Our formal psychology as such is less than a hundred years old, and so represents a recent version of an endeavor probably as old as human history. It is also the product of European and American culture, society, and intellectual history, and as such is only one of innumerable *psychologies* [though for us by far the most familiar and comfortable] which have been articulated as an implicit or explicit part of the fabric of reality in every culture, past and present. [40]

A more careful look at the import of this broader view of the psychological, or, as earlier expressed, metaphysical, interests of humankind will guide the concluding remarks of this thesis in our final chapters. Here I have in mind to note that current psychotherapy is both relatively young – as pointed out above – and all too commonly assumed to have had its birth with Freud and those who followed; those who diverted. Yet for our purposes here, the smaller historical perspective is appropriate. It highlights what has been our focus in this chapter and keeps our attention on more secular, recent understandings of both therapist and therapy, as this chapter concludes in an effort to define and describe precisely these more recent understandings.

Corsini et. al. begin their historical grouping of psychotherapies with Freud [1856–1939]. The next grouping is that of Adlerian Individual Psychotherapy [Alfred Adler 1870–1937], and then that of Analytical Depth Psychology as typified by its pioneer, Carl Gustav Jung [1875-1961]. Let me elucidate here some basic points of departure as early thinkers and colleagues of Sigmund Freud began charting broader perspectives on psychology and human development.

Remembering the medical model that eventually took hold and which exerted strong influence, especially during the period covered by the catalogue of psychotherapies listed above, I draw attention here to a discernable tension between Freud and some of his early followers. Doctors Freud and Jung actually met frequently in Vienna to discuss and create foundational theories which became the basis for psychoanalysis. However, Jung eventually separated from Freud. The year is generally placed at about 1913. [41] Their *Wednesday Society* fell into both arguments and eventual disagreements – largely over issues of personality structure.

Early in the twentieth century, discussions and disagreement -- now by letters -- began to center on the issue of pathology: Whether those with conflicts, concerns, issues or life problems were framed in pathology, or whether some larger view – and therefore larger treatment modality – needed formulation in order to accommodate the complexities of a persons seeking to understand, and be in a healthy relationship with, their inner and outer worlds.

We find good evidence of this in the scholarly historical works of those who tracked and recorded early discussions between Freud and Jung. We also find the same material presented through a different, comparative, lens by those who charted and compared the theoretical starting point of these two major theorists – both concerned with human development and its complexity. While Freud grounded such complexity in libidinal sources attached to a mythological interpretation seeming to underline parent-child, as well as sexual, conflict, Jung et. al. moved to a larger myth and a wider lens. Far from an unscientific opiate, argued Jung, religious and spiritual sensibilities on the part of both doctor and patient – part, simply, of a philosophical anthropology – needed a place in the healing equation.

In 1910, Freud insisted on appointing Jung Permanent President of the International Psychoanalytic Society and asked him to promise *never to abandon the sexual theory. That is the most essential thing of all. You see, we must make a dogma out of it, an unshakable bulwark.* Jung asked him, *A bulwark against what?* and was told that sexual theory would be a bulwark *against the black tide of mud* which was *occultism.* What Freud meant by *occultism* was everything dear to Jung's heart – philosophy, religion and mysticism. It seemed to Jung that Freud has lost his scientific objectivity and was descending into ideology. [42]

Those interested in the subject can pursue commentaries that shed further light on the personal and professional, including scientific, struggles that eventually led to the final break between Freud and Jung which followed Jung's publication of his book *Psychology of the Unconscious* [later revised and called *Symbols of Transformation*]. [43] Here I return to scholars of comparative psychological theories equipped to tease out for us what I see as the beginnings of that wider lens in both understanding, and treating, client-patients.

Noting systemic, theoretical starting points in the perspectives which both flowed, and departed, from valuable Freudian insights, Mosak [44] identifies several differences with Freudian theory which present themselves in Adlerian Individual Psychology. Recall that both Adler and Jung were studious colleagues of Freud. Yet Adler, already having his own established practice, demonstrated theoretical convictions born of experience, research and practice. As Mosak points out, this allegedly first challenge to Freudian theory required attention to the subjective as well as the objective; a wider look at social dimensions of health instead of presuming a physiological etiology; Freud's views on causality vs. Adler's et. al. inclusion of teleology [τέλος Gk. *end or purpose*] of human functioning, including distress; the reductionistic structure of Freud's views of the human personality; Adler's view that *parts* -- memory, emotions, behavior – are in the service of the whole individual; and, finally, for our purposes; the centering of Freud's constructs around the intrapsychic, the *intra*personal, as distinguished from the broader view of Adlerian psychology which argued that ...*man can only be understood* **inter***personally, a social being moving through and interacting with his environment.* [45]

What, then, of Jung and his parallel departure from Freud? It is important to note that, like Adler, C. G. Jung reached beyond pathologies whose etiologies were presumed to point the way to treatment and cure. It can be argued that while both Adler and Jung prized and captured, albeit in different ways and to different degrees, the phenomenological, experiential material presented by a troubled client in the consulting room, both of these analytical psychologists not only embraced the subjective, but also remained open to categories of human experience which did not fit neatly into pathological tendencies [*etiologies*] seemingly so necessary for a Freudian diagnosis.

The charted comparison in Mosak's work helps us to visualize where a broadening of the theoretical framework began: attention to the subjective as well as the objective; inclusion of social -- including, for Jung, the cultural, historical, philosophical-religious -- over against merely the physiological substrata; working with a whole individual rather than focusing on a division into the various parts of the person/ality; an interpersonal perspective on assessment and therefore on healing, therapeutic relationships.

For his part, Jung seemed unable, and later consciously unwilling, to put aside his passionate interest in history, mythology, literature and religious ideation when it came to his own writings, his laboratory research and his consulting room. Like Adler, he valued Freud's scientific approach and cogent theoretical framework. Yet from his own experience, as well as contact with patients in his capacity as clinician in training, and later as professional practitioner, Carl Jung was beset by the depth and mystery of human consciousness. While research and theories around mechanisms of repression had indeed piqued Freud's early interest in Jung's work, such mechanistic, reductionistic, physiological explanations of how and why psychic material moved between levels of consciousness seemed too narrow. Like Adler, though we find no evidence of their direct debate and dialogue over the matter, Jung was drawn more to the *gestalt*, the whole person, and the environmental space within and around humankind. Eventually Jung appropriated the notion of an even larger source of experience beyond what Freud had accommodated within his intrapsychic formulations.

Known for the attention he gave to dreams as potent symbols of this larger source of experience, Jung took the position that symbols disclosed aspects of the psyche which, when brought to consciousness, held great power and evidenced archetypal material akin to what we will later understand in the context of spiritual hungers. While not entirely separate from cognition and intellectual functioning, the mere processing or analysis of issues flowing into the awake consciousness may miss much of what the psyche is telling both analyst and patient. In the framework of depth psychology, symbolic material cried out for both expression and amplification, and not simply interpretation. Rather than merely noted and then connected to conscious materials by analysis, symbolic material is welcomed by Jungians and given wide parameters in which to roam.

Dreams are but one example of these powerful symbols which invite both therapist and patient into mythical constellations of the self. Symbols evidence the mysterious nature of human consciousness and point to a source definition of humanity itself. Symbols, for Jung, arise because of the symbolic nature of life itself, as well as the human capacity for creativity as the self reaches mysteriously for healing. As Whitmont has pointed out, ...*it was Jung's concern, and indeed the very point of departing with Freud, to show that intuition and emotion and the capacity to apperceive and create by way of symbols are basic modes of human functioning, no less so than perception through the sense organs and through thinking.* [46]

Jung's psychological theory not only gathered to itself a totality of human experience known to the individual, but also the symbolic value of all human experience – conscious or not – and used such language in piecing together an analytical approach to therapy that made no apology for its reference to symbol and myth. Even the occult, for Carl

Jung, was reframed and valued as part of the human story – as it was part of his own.

For Jung, myth was essential to the human race. To live without a myth that explains the cosmos, our place in it and how we are to live our lives was to be *uprooted*. Without myth, we would have no link to past or present. To understand ourselves we need to understand the myths that had formed our civilizations. Individual consciousness was *only the flower and the fruit of a season, sprung from the perennial rhizome beneath the earth; and it would find itself in better accord with the truth if it took the existence of the rhizome into its calculations. For the root matter is the mother of all things.* [47]

Through his study of myth, Jung came to a deeper appreciation of its function for individuals who presented themselves to him for analysis; he also sensed from comparative religious studies that myth, and what it disclosed, provided a map to a greater, foundational, cross-cultural set of stories which he deemed symbolic at the archetypal level. He began formulating an idea radical to medical science at the time: that of a human group mind, the collective unconscious.

This was a shift from the from a psychology which saw each individual's psyche as made up solely of his or her own past history to a vision of humankind as having a 'group mind' which was the inheritance of all. In this new psychology, there was a role for spirituality. [48]

Whether analyst in the sense of these early post-Freudian perspectives, or therapist in more contemporary psycho-social contexts, psychological health and its modalities of healing were not to be confined, at least for all, to narrow, reductionistic categories of human development any more than physician-healers of the body can escape inquiry into the so called mind-body connection. Professionals enter into a counselor-client relationship with honed skills appropriate to their vocation; the trust given them is a thinly veiled request to see the whole person even as they apply their therapeutic methods in ways consistent with their professional goals.

The work of psychological healing, the task of therapy, moved beyond identifiable pathology – at least in the analytical, gestalt and other constructs loosely gathered into the transpersonal schools – and entered the arena of human experience: The whole person as patient; the person as part of a larger community and a larger history; the here-and-now appreciated as part of a larger, on-going story; myth seen as connecting a particular culture's meaning system to that of another culture, another time, a parallel effort to understand and interpret ones world of experience.

The implications for possible definitions of therapist and what a therapist does, however comprehensive, are nonetheless decidedly shaped by the presenting seeker's problem as well as the therapist-healer's particular training, perspective and theory-based skills. We have mentioned earlier that some will emphasize heavily the educational aspects of counseling [cognitive, psycho-educational, rational-emotive]; other will have an eye to intrapsychic conflicts which present themselves [psychoanalytic]; still others will concentrate on changing behavior – as in addiction counseling, which is usually combined with psycho-educational, cognitive and group process approaches. The emphases are varied; often they are applied eclectically, depending on the expressed need of the client and the coexisting problems brought to the counselor-client relationship. Yet foundational to any therapeutic process within the framework we have circumscribed in these pages, and therefore central to the identity and role of the therapist, is the work of *psychotherapy* as described by Roger Walsh:

> Psychotherapy is a planned, emotionally charged, confiding interaction between a trained, socially sanctioned healer and a sufferer. During this interaction the healer seeks to relieve the sufferer's distress and disability through symbolic interventions, primarily words but also sometimes bodily activities. The healer may or may not involve the patient's relatives and others in the healing rituals. Psychotherapy also often includes helping the patient to accept and endure suffering as an inevitable aspect of life that can be used as an opportunity for personal growth...All psychotherapeutic methods elaborations and variations of age-old procedures of psychological healing. [49]

Typical of holistic approaches to therapy representing the analytical, *depth psychology* perspective is what Hillman points out when he views the client-patient as fundamentally a *mystery*. Adopting this therapeutic stance, I believe, takes nothing away from other categories of understanding human personality and its developmental theories. Rather, it is a foundational perspective, an attitude; one that holds the client-patient in the kind of awe which reminds the therapist that the client is not his to create or control. Still valuing individual theories and techniques meant to operationalize a therapeutic relationship and enhance the well-being of the client, sensing the mystery of a whole person sitting before you reminds the therapist that this is indeed a privileged work, a lofty goal and a calling long known to history.

The person who comes to counseling comes to be freed from the oppression with accidents, to find truth by stepping clean out of banalities which he himself recognizes as such but is obsessively trapped within. The task is to leap qualitatively into the unknown...The longer and better one knows another, as in analysis... the less one can say for sure about the true root of the trouble, since the true root is always the person himself and the person is neither a disease nor a problem, but fundamentally an insoluble mystery. [50]

Part VI – Conclusion

Our location of the therapist as healer lies within the a psychological framework more akin to post Freudian schools if only in appropriating to the therapist's goal both intrapsychic and interpersonal issues and experience. Recent developments in system approaches, for example conjoint and structural family therapies, heighten our awareness that threads from every significant, formative person in the patient's life enters the office with him. Yet long before Family Therapy's coming of age, theorist-practitioners like Adler and Jung welcomed both the interior and external worlds of a patient's psyche. The welcoming is marked by empathy and the challenge for the therapist to empathize with the client while strategically managing a genuine, yet still professional, relationship. Hillman often speaks of this as a conscious decision on the part of the analyst to create space within himself in order to *feel into* his client. Such a conscious decision on the part of therapist is both preparation for a healing encounter as well as an act of docility to one's call as a healer.

> *Empathy* comes to us as a translation of the word of the German psychologists, 'einfulung' which means literally 'feeling into.' It is derived from the Greek 'pathos,' meaning a deep and strong feeling akin to suffering, prefixed with the preposition 'in.' The parallel with the 'sympathy' is obvious. But whereas sympathy denotes 'feeling with' and may lead into sentimentality, empathy means a much deeper state of identification of personalities in which one person so feels himself into the other as to temporarily lose his own identity. It is in this profound and somewhat mysterious process of empathy that understanding, influence, and the other significant relations between persons take place. [51]

While honoring Freud's pioneering work in intrapsychic phenomena and pathology, I understand and define a therapist's identity, and therefore the implied professional goal, as a professional who understands health from the perspective of the World Health Organization's definition: *...as optimal functioning ... not only as internal harmony and consistency of functioning within the organism, but also the capacity of the organism to maintain itself in its environment – especially in the human case to extend itself creatively to an ever expanding culture. ... As health is a state of complete physical, mental and social well-being and not merely the absence of disease or infirmity,* [52] it follows that the therapist-healer's attention will be drawn to all manner of presenting problems to attain a healthy understanding of, and creative relationship to, both the internal and external *worlds* of clients.

Whether a therapist's training has sharpened his psychoanalytic, depth psychological, cognitive-behavioral, rational-emotive or myriad other professional orientations, the client should be seen as an individual with a unique history as well as someone participating in a larger world within and around him.

Adler recognizes empathy as one of the creative functions in personality and goes on to say

Empathy occurs in the moment one human being speaks with another. It is impossible to understand another individual if it is impossible at the same time to identify one's self with him... If we seek for the origin of this ability to act and feel as if we were someone else, we can find it in the inborn social feeling. This is, as a matter of fact, a cosmic feeling and a reflection of the connectedness of the whole cosmos which lives in us, it is an inescapable characteristic of being human. [53]

Jung uses the image or notion of the therapist and patient merging in such a way that each is changed.

The meeting of two personalities is like the contact of two chemical substances; if there is any reaction, both are transformed. We should expect the doctor to have an influence on the patient in every effective psychic treatment; but this influence can only take place when he, too, is affected by the patient. [54]

In my own years of counseling practice spanning both religious and secular settings, the debate about professional boundaries between counselor and client, therapist and patient, has been alive and well. The therapeutic value of maintaining professional distance as a counselor never, in my hearing, suggested a lack of concern or of empathy. Today, there is even more caution being exercised in this regard out of liability concerns in an increasingly litigious climate. I maintain that an empathetic posture, or, in the words of Karl Rogers, an *unconditional positive regard* is meant to underscore a non-judgmental attitude on the part of the therapist, rather than a caviler attitude about one's role as counselor. Recall that one of the traits of a professional is that of adhering to professionally acknowledged standards in practice. These standards, created from a vision of both the lofty goals of the profession as well as practical formulations of resulting behavior, serve the counselor-client relationship in ways meant to foster trust, allow empathy, preserve appropriate professional practice and yield improved quality of living for the client.

Moreover, it is the self-awareness of the therapist around the goals of his freely chosen profession which give proper meaning to boundaries and inform appropriate practice. The well-being of the client is primary, even as Hillman has helped us to understand that a therapist's call cannot be fulfilled without the client's pain. Both are in the room, and, from an analytical perspective, both should expect to be changed. Of the many ways, then, of understanding what and who a therapist *is*, a crucial first step is to have the therapist explore and embrace an acceptable definition of therapist. In Jungian terms, and since definitions are expansive in his writings, a therapist might be encouraged to understand the myths that shape him as person and professional. In the words of Hillman,

> ...according to individual art and style – which in turn derive from the individual myth lived into by each analyst – a variety of models of practice are offered: Some are high priests of the cult of the soul, or its confessors or directors; others are shepherds of souls, group leaders; some are politicians, sophists, educators; some are pragmatists, practical advisors, or biologists minutely examining life history; some are nursing mothers encouraging growth, inspirers, or confidants; still other may be a 'mystes' or 'epoptes', a shaman, an initiator, or a guru of the body, awakening its sensitivity. [55]

Hillman's language and style do not typify that found in journals of Western Psychology. Yet this short reflection on the multiple myths of self-awareness among analysts is remarkable if one thinks about the settings in which therapists find themselves working. With such a broad range of self-directing identities informing a variety of therapists whose common connection might be found in the general profile of the professionals who do this healing work, what can be said about who they are beyond persons of professional empathy? Presuming therapists have been trained, recognized for their qualifications and commissioned to practice, what joins them in a common professional identity?

The movement of my thesis in some way begs that question. Beyond training and technique – necessary and worthy of any professional practice – there dwells the larger myth of meaning, purpose and guidance within the therapeutic setting: humankind's connection to, and thirst for, a greater love, power and presence captured by the perennial search for a *wholly other* realm of experience: *Spirituality*. That is the subject of the next chapter as it appears in notions surrounding the *priestly* healer.

One last characteristic of the therapist is the feeling of freedom. Needing no specific religious reference, therapeutic assumptions and beliefs about human freedom not only give space within us for health and well-being, but also frame the myth of both seeker and healer as they enter into a therapeutic relationship. With freedom comes consequent responsibility.

> The psychotherapist Otto Rank has definitively explained the importance of freedom and responsibility in psychotherapy. Long one of Freud's closest associates, Rank was finally forced to break with the master because of Freud's refusal to admit the centrality of creative will in psychoanalytic treatment. Rank holds that in the long last we must admit that the individual creates his own personality by creative willing, and that neurosis is due precisely to the fact that the patient cannot will constructively.
>
> It is possible to grow in freedom. The more mentally healthy the person becomes, the more his is able to mold creatively the materials of life, and hence the more he has appropriated his potentiality of freedom. When the counselor, therefore, helps the counselee to overcome his personality difficulty, he has actually helped him to become more free. To summarize our first principle of personality,

freedom, in the form of a guide for counseling: *it is the function of the counselor to lead the counselee to acceptance of responsibility for the conduct and outcome of his life.* The counselor will show him how deep lie the roots of decision, how all previous experience and the forces of the unconscious must be reckoned with; but in the end he will aid the counselee to appropriate and use his possibilities of freedom. [56]

Chapter Two Notes

[23] Atkinson, Donald T.: *Magic, Myth and Medicine* [1956] The World Publishing Company, NY pg. 21

[24] ibid.

[25] ibid.

[26] Marty, Martin E. & Vaux, Kenneth L., [ed.]: *Health/Medicine and the Faith Traditions* [1982] Fortress Press, Philadelphia pg. 53

[27] Atkinson, Op. Cit., Pg. 38

[28] ibid.

[29] Miller, op. cit., pg. 12

[30] ibid., pg. 4

[31] ibid.

[32] ibid. pg. 6

[33] Ashley and O'Rourke, op. cit., pg. 99

[34] ibid., pg. 86

[35] ibid., pg. 100

[36] ibid., pg. 101

[37] ibid., pg. 96

[38] ibid., pg. 97

[39] Corsini, Raymond J. et. al. *Current Psychotherapies* [1979] F. E. Peacock Publishers Inc., Itasca, Illinois, pg. x

[40] Macquarrie, John: *Paths In Spirituality* [1992] Morehouse Publishing, Harrisburg, PA pg. 18

[41] Crowley, Vivianne: *Jungian Spirituality* [1998] Thorsons, Harper Collins Publishers, London pg. 16

[42] ibid., pg. 15

[43] ibid.

[44] Corsini, op. cit., pg. 49

[45] ibid.

[46] Whitmont, Edward C.: *The Symbolic Quest* [1960] Princeton University Press, Princeton, NJ, pg. 18
[47] Crowley, op. cit., pg. 16
[48] ibid., pg. 16
[49] Walsh, op. cit., 184
[50] Hillman, In Search, pg. 26
[51] May, Rollo: *The Art of Counseling* [1967] Abingdon Press, NY, pg. 75
[52] Ashley and O'Rourke, op. cit., pg. 25
[53] May, op. cit., pg. 79
[54] ibid.
[55] Hillman, op. cit., Myth, pg. 17
[56] May, op. cit., pSg. 53

Chapter Three
Priest as Healer

I was already a Roman Catholic seminarian during my college years in the late 1960's. My life consisted of studies, side employment and an abiding aspiration to be a *priest*. As the Roman Catholic seminary process was undergoing huge changes after many decades of a seamless, predictable older style of preparation within separate seminary walls, we felt like pioneers blazing a new trail. Houses of study were formed on local college campuses. We were assimilated into their academic programs while living in a separate campus community held together by prayer, meals and a spirit of fraternity. While new experiences were happening all around us, each June during those four years we traveled to the cathedral to witness the ordination of those who were our seniors in the theologate — the *major seminary*.

My memory of those rites is vivid. They were motivational and inspiring. As Hippocrates encouraged his early followers to engage the desire of the patient to be well, these rites, by their nature, had a kind of power to engage the desire to be holy. While I will say more about the *power of symbol* later, let me say here that if there is truth in the theory that experiences that bring many levels of sensory experience to the fore are those most vividly remembered, those ordination ceremonies advance that conclusion very well.

The music – both Latin chant and English polyphony — was rich; the cathedral pews were filled with family and friends awaiting this great day in the life of their sons, brothers, uncles, friends. Everyone assisting in the sanctuary seemed to have not only a different role, but a unique *vestment* marking their ritual duties. The odor of incense filled the air amidst the bright portable lights of television cameras from local stations; flashbulbs from the pews flickered and punctuated the solemn proclamations of sacred scripture. This indeed was *Haec dies. Jubilate Deo!* In the middle of this solemn ceremony where men had processed through our midst to the altar, the ordaining bishop solemnly and without words placed his hands on the head of each of the *ordinands* kneeling before him. Prior to that moment, they had lain prostrate on the great marble floor in front of the main altar as the entire congregation invoked the prayers of the church. The whole church was asked to grace these men -- those who had died and were thought of as the *church* triumphant, as well as those present and still struggling in this *valley of tears*. The Litany of the Saints rang out in antiphonal rhythm between cantor and congregation, begging the prayers of all for these men and the ministry that lay before them.

After each man was ordained through the *invocation of the Holy Spirit and the laying on of [the Bishop's] hands*, all ordained priests present came forward and placed his hands on each of the new priests' heads. As this seemingly endless procession of vested priests moved from one newly ordained to the next, the choir led the congregation in the traditional chant which invoked the *Holy Spirit: Veni Creator Spiritus.*

> *Veni Creator Spiritus; Mentes tuorum visita.*
> Come, Holy Spirit. Dwell in us.

Most memorable for me, however, was the investiture of each new priest. It is also an image I invoke as I begin this chapter on the priestly healer. For just minutes before, these men were *deacons*. They held a different, however transitory, *order* or position in the church. The sign of their office was a *stole* placed over a single shoulder and clasped at their side.

As the company of ordaining clergy melded back into the congregation after imposing their hands, each new priest removed his diaconal stole and was vested in kind and style with that of priest. Even more eye-catching was the placement on each man of the priestly chasuble, a kind of large tunic draped over the font and back of the man-now-priest. And while it no longer takes place in the ordination rites of my tradition, this last, larger vestment remained tied at the top and back of each priest like a roman shade that had been dropped down fully in front but remained up, and open, in the back. It was only when the power and authority of their priestly office was ritually and fully passed on to each new priest that the remaining portion of the vestment was lowered. A gradual, symbolic procession of its own as the *powers* and *duties* of his new office were themselves unfolded within each priestly soul.

The time was indeed the 1960's and the ritual, by then, was celebrated in English rather than the older Latin. The image obviously references a particular tradtion within Christianity, as well as a specific time wherein the ritual did not yet fully reflect that tradition's renewed understandings of either priesthood or ministry. The remembered symbolism of that decade can not only be traced to a mystical theology of who a priest was and the sacred duties handed down, I would argue that those rituals capture some of the pivotal aspects of priestly identity and function which survive both that time and that particular tradition.

Forgive sin. Bless and consecrate. Offer sacrifice in the name of the people. Anoint the sick and dying with chrism, and bring them sacred *unction.* Teach and preach the Holy Scriptures. Care for God's people.

It all happened during a long, richly symbolic ceremony with roots deep in both its own denominational life and touching upon rituals spawned outside even its own religious tradition. These men, once just a part of the community, had been set aside for sacred duties. Their hands had been anointed to bless and heal; their hearts were to draw life from the sustenance of a *holy spirit*; their frail human nature was to be fed with the saving Word of God; their mission required them to *shake loose* [*βαπτίζω* {Gk. 'to shake loose; 'baptize'}] the bonds of sin and its slavery to self; they were being ordained and sent to bring living water to insatiable, thirsty souls. Theirs would be a mission of *healing*, largely through the ministry of helping people in their care to be *reconciled* to God and to one another. Acknowledging the particular historical and denominational context of our example, the documents of Vatican II concerning the *Ministry and Life of Priests* are thematically helpful in considering the task of unity and reconciliation.

> ...priests have been placed in the midst of the laity so that they may lead them all to the unity of charity, 'loving one another with brotherly affection; outdoing one another in sharing honor' [Rom. 12:10]. Theirs is the task, then, of bringing about agreement among divergent outlooks in such a way that nobody may feel a stranger in the Christian community. They are at once to be defenders of the common good... [57]

During those early years of my life and my own aspirations toward ministry, I may not have understood much beyond the symbolic, mystical identity and duties of those being *set apart* during a ceremony which left vivid traces of its polyvalent ritual. I certainly could not have pondered then the practical ways by which these men were to take their place in a church which saw itself as being *in the world, but not of it.* Intuitively and visually, however, I knew that they now wore the mantle of priest and had taken to themselves a spiritual, healing role among us. Later I would also understand that men and women called to ministry in other traditions were also ordained or otherwise publicly recognized as being set apart to serve within either a specifically religious, or generally spiritual, context.

The communities that sent them may have had differing theologies and rituals shaping their place and duties within congregations. Yet all recognized, blessed and sent them. Priests, ministers, rabbis and others were sent forth with a message founded in spiritual truths and commissioned to teach, sanctify and heal those seekers and communities who would embrace their touch. On that day in my memory, and at some level of ritual impact, I sensed these men left the cathedral as *priestly leaders and healers.* I would later have that suspicion confirmed through experience. I would begin to understand on my own some of the essential elements which attend all manner of spiritual guides across a variety of contexts and throughout various chapters of history. As in the previous chapter where I chose the term *therapist* to enfold those healing from a more secular, psychological perspective, *priest* will serve in this chapter to connote those who avail themselves of theological and spiritual wisdom traditions as they make themselves available for the work of healing.

I invoke this moment from my past, therefore, in order to begin a task in this chapter that eschews the confines of words. As a high church ordination appeals to a variety of signs, symbols and senses to unfold the mysterious role of priest, so the priest not only lives in, but also appeals to and employs, the metaphysical in carrying out the work to which she is called.

By the time I took my place as priest within the same tradition [1973], liturgical and theological renewal had begun following Vatican II's attention to the *Church in the Modern World.* The basic rites of ordination remained the same; however the last vestiges of sacred aloofness between priest and God's people were wearing thin. The newer ordination ritual replaced the drama of a passion play with the joy of selfless service. I had been among the people of the parish where I was ordained for a year by the time I was called to priestly orders. The attempt was to have the people know the person, and to commend him with their own voice to the ordaining bishop.

At several levels of liturgical renewal, the Roman Catholic Church was moving toward aspects of a preparation and ordination process which many of the reformers envisioned, and which many Protestant denominations had adopted as standard decades ago. But for us, there was a freshness to the changes; so too was there a theology in the documents of Vatican II which encouraged them. The inherent mission and message in these rituals however, like others which set aside persons to treasure and employ spiritual gifts, remained the same: Be in the world, but tread lightly; go forth with eyes, ears and heart set on a larger, spiritual reality.

Priests can learn, by brotherly and friendly association with each other and with other people, to cultivate human values and appreciate crated *creatd* goods as gifts of God. While living in the world they should still realize that according to the Word of our Lord and Master they are not of the world. By using the world, then, as those who do not use it they will come to that liberty by which they will be freed from all inordinate anxiety and will become docile to the divine voice in their daily life. From this liberty and docility grows that spiritual insight through which is found a right attitude to the world and to early goods. [58]

I have employed a personal memory from a specific time and tradition for two reasons. First, it captures a particular expression of an ordination ritual wherein ceremonial parts unfolded in ways which make explicit a few, key understandings of the identity and role of a designated minister-priest as expressed within several of the Christian traditions. Second, it provides the writer with a familiar base from which to enlarge the notion of priest to other religious and spiritual frameworks.

The remembered image, and the gradual transfer of power and duties highlighted in the unfolding of the new *Father's* chasuble, disclosed priestly aspects of role and function reminiscent of those captured by John Morgan in his book *Scholar, Priest, and Pastor*. Utilizing for a moment Morgan's *litany of descriptive words* [59] for the priestly category of clergy, it is clear to me that both older and contemporary rites of ordination in the Roman Catholic tradition identify these aspects of role-identity, among others: liturgy; sacraments; Eucharist; confession, absolution; divine economy. For purposes of a departure point upon which I will build a larger framework supporting thematic aspects of a *priestly* identity, let me first refer to Morgan's categories and their meaning.

The priestly functions of the clergy are categorized into five identifiable activities, namely, 1) the leading of public worship, 2) presiding over Holy Communion, 3) discharging functions of ministry that are defined as *sacramental*, yet other than Communion, 4) functioning as a spiritual director or advisor ... and, finally, 5) exercising discipline by way of enforcing the canons of the denomination on errant members of the community. [60]

In the Roman Catholic denominational setting, explicit charges were given to the ordained relating to each category above. In Morgan's study, and in his application of a *social construction of reality* approach to the four Christian denominations he surveyed, the working assumption is that any of these categories of priestly functioning have a potential place in the self-understanding of at least Roman Catholic, Lutheran, Methodist and Episcopal clergy.

While we may use several of these particular aspects of the categories of *priestly* identity and functioning cited and used by John Morgan, our discussion of the *priest as healer* in a larger context will gravitate around the work of *priest* as experienced in the healing dimensions of liturgy inclusive of worship, sacrament including ritual, and spiritual guide as an aspect of Morgan's discipline-based *divine economy*. Note that these focused areas are but a few among many available to the priest-healer. Note also that I use Morgan's general priestly categories as a convenient departure point for activities germane to priest and not to suggest his meanings or interpretation.

Before proceeding, let me note again that the thesis moves toward establishing the spiritual dimensions of any therapeutic relationship. This chapter is intended to highlight several pivotal aspects of healing as they are expressed by, and captured within, those who sense and accept a vocation to a specifically spiritual context for that work. I use the term *priest* as primary referent for such persons and their activity. Moreover, since any one of these chapters could be a thesis standing alone, the work of Chapter Three is necessarily only as expansive as it must be to substantiate and inform the chapters that follow. Themes presented here will appear in the work that follows, work that is meant to advance the conclusion as stated in the introduction: ... *a therapeutic relationship, fully and rightly understood, and whether consciously referenced or not, rests fundamentally on spiritual foundations.*

Part I –Inherent Suppositions: Philosophical Anthropology; Theological Anthropology

Vocatus atque non vocatus, Deus adherit.
- From the Oracle at Delphi

Some authors translate the above quotation as *"Called or not called, the God is there."* Latin grammar would also allow the rendering *"Named or not, God is present."* In either case, we are reminded of how an implicit spiritual perspective, while open to explicit theological discourse, can capture a foundational anthropological perspective which includes the whole of our experience as humans. It is possible to frame all of reality as imbued with the sacred, and thus even beg the question related to those perennial dualistic categories of *human and divine, sacred and profane, matter and form, material and spiritual* and so on.

Carl Jung, who once asserted that any psychological question was at once a spiritual question, had the above Latin inscription carved into the stone above the doorway to his home in Kusnacht. His anthropological perspective disclosed this sort of spiritual foundation. *For Jung, myth was now the key to understanding the human psyche. He was no longer interested in individual psychology so much as the psyche of the whole human race – its dreams, myths and visions, and the religious and spiritual traditions that express them.* [61]

A philosophical anthropology that embraces more than material reality is at the very least *spiritual*. Conceptualizations of God, the sacred, the divine or the holy which are seen as natural to that reality [world view] may move a philosophical anthropology, generically *spiritual*, into a more specifically *theological* hermeneutic. While this and the following chapters may make reference to images of a *deity* appropriated by certain religions or cultures, the view of reality being employed here as a grounding assumption is that of a broad, underlying philosophical perspective on our world and the life which inhabits it. That perspective is best described in Rudolf Otto's *The Idea of the Holy*; it is his insightful conceptualization of the *numinous* that frames the work of this chapter.

> Holiness – the holy – is a category of interpretation and valuation peculiar to the sphere of religion. … While it is complex, it contain a quite specific element or 'moment,' which sets it apart from 'the rational' in the meaning we gave to that word, and which remains inexpressible – an __*αρρητον*__ or 'ineffabile' – in the sense that it completely eludes apprehension in terms of concepts. …
> It will be our endeavor to suggest this unnamed Something to the reader as far as we may, so that he may himself feel it. There is no religion in which it does not live as the innermost core, and without it no religious would be worthy of the name. It is pre-eminently a living force in the Semitic religions… Here, too, it has a nature of its own, viz. the Hebrew _qadosh_, to which the Greek _ἁγιός_ and the Latin 'sanctus,' and, more accurately still, 'sacer,' are the corresponding terms.
> Accordingly, it is worth while, as we have said, to find a word to stand for this element in isolation, this 'extra' in the meaning of 'holy' above and beyond the meaning of goodness. … For this reason I adopt a word coined from the Latin 'numen.' 'Omen' has given us 'ominous,' and there is no reason why from 'numen' we should not similarly for a word 'numinous.'
> I shall speak, then, of a unique 'numinous' category of value found wherever the category is applied. The mental state is *sui generis* and irreducible to any other; and, therefore, like every

absolutely primary and elementary datum, while it admits of being discussed, it cannot be strictly defined.

Cannot you now realize for yourself what it is? In other words our X cannot, strictly speaking, be taught, it can only be evoked, awakened in the mind; as everything that comes 'of the spirit' must be awakened. [62]

At the end of the ordination ceremony to which I referred above, the choir burst forth in the hymn *Ecce Sacerdos Magnus.* A biblical reference to Christ the High priest, it nonetheless captured the identity and mission handed over to those newly ordained priests. Even with a marked change in the theological stance of that tradition as it reverted to the holiness of all God's people, the mystery of the ordination ritual concluded with a visual and musical expression of the *sacred.* For regardless of efficacy, or of the mechanisms and the persons by which people and life itself were transformed in *holiness,* the *sacred* was presupposed as unquestionably available to human persons just as the potential to *be seen as holy* [imago dei] already dwelt within the potential for communion with the divine.

Within such an anthropological perspective, where sacredness is both immanent and transcendent, where the divine can be named and worshipped in a religious context or remains completely ineffable, but awakened, we return our attention to *priest as healer.*

Liturgy = The work a The people

— The priest's work

Part II – Ritual and Liturgical Dimensions

The Greek root of *liturgy* [_λειτουργέια_] encompasses more than religious ceremony and ritual practice. It quite literally connotes the *work* that one does. For the healer-priest, I argue that any activity which takes place in the specific context of the *ministry* to which a priest is called is, then, his *work.* Furthermore, other religious or spiritual healers who exercise their spiritual ministrations in a conscious, professed way – and who do so marked by the general counselor-client relationship qualities previously discussed – engage in a *liturgy.* Such activity, or spiritual work, belongs not only to their identity as priest-healers, but is an extension of it.

The work by Morgan, cited above, applied several categories of ministry to four denominational traditions in Christian ministry. Each category described one of several expressions, or works, of Christian ministry. Each had the potential of application to a Roman Catholic, Methodist, Lutheran or Episcopal minister's self-understanding of an aspect of his ministry – his *liturgy* – being applied in various degrees to the categories used in the research tool, i.e. being *scholar, priest or pastor.* While Dr. Morgan rightly included the leading of public worship, including presiding at Communion, within the category of *priestly* functions as he approached his study, here the meaning of the word *liturgy* is a more general characterization of all of the healing *work* that a *priest* might perform out of the context of a spiritual identity and mission.

Although there are subtle distinctions between *liturgy* and *worship* not requiring elaboration for our work here, one aspect of liturgy, a form of it, is indeed worship. To the degree that a spiritual healer leads, facilitates or creates opportunities for worship, he is not only faithful to one aspect of his commission as *priest,* but, and more explicitly, he invites individuals and communities to a deeper level of

73

awareness and participation in communion with the very source of the sacred. In the Christian perspective, Macquarrie expresses it this way.

> Paul enunciates a kind of law: *Whatever a man sows, that he will also reap* ... This surely brings us close to the meaning of worship, considered in its manward aspects as a discipline...
>
> This is the work of God, the *opus Dei,* in St. Benedict's phrase. True worship is work, though one might hardly think this if one has in mind the conventional worship of many Christian churches. It is, furthermore, work which issues in the most valuable results. ... To be sure, this is not *productive work,* as the economist understands it. It is not work that adds anything to the gross national product. But, more importantly, it is *creative* work. It is creating persons of spiritual depth, and through them the creative Spirit will reach out further still.[63]

It is difficult to overstate the dimensions of healing that reside in any of the ritual, liturgical or worship experiences to which the priest invites both individuals and communities given to his care. Once grounded in a worldview where the boundaries between the sacred and the profane create more experiential overlap than rational separation, any human *inclinatio ad cautelum* [cf. Thomas Aquinas, the *disposition toward praise {of God}*] can be understood as an entirely natural response to conscious awareness of spiritual power and presence in life itself.

> We have called faith an *existential attitude,* and orientation of the whole man, and when we talk about the *religious man* we mean the man who is characterized by this attitude or orientation. ... we tried to do justice to the initiative of the holy in

awakening faith, but we felt it necessary also to show that man is so constituted that the quest for faith belongs to the very structure of his existence. This does not mean that man is *naturally religious*, but it does recognize a continuity between man's quest for wholeness and selfhood, and the divine activity in grace and revelation. This is far from making religion a human activity, but it does recognize a root of religion in human existence. [64]

Whether in the context of a religious tradition wherein the divine is named and described in human language, or found among those whose worldview is marked by a conscious belief in an ineffable Spirit, the human response to the sacred is a connection which can heal. Inviting a person or community to worship can take many forms as the priest-healer's *liturgy of a spiritual life* draws another to deeper awareness of its sacred character. The human quest for wholeness and selfhood, once seen as belonging to an existence fundamentally oriented to communion with the source of life itself, can be approached and strengthened in times of prayer, reflection, contemplation, joyful praise or, indeed, any insight gained during spiritual guidance which leads to worshipful acknowledgement of its spiritual source. It is the priest-healer's privileged role and holy place among us that allows the kind of healing which flows from a progressively more free, conscious and intentional embrace of the sacred by those seeking to become whole.

... worship is a work leading to intangible results of the highest value for the quality of human life, and it is to be hoped that there will always be some people who, not for themselves alone, but for the whole Church and for all mankind, will devote themselves to the *opus Dei*. ... must we not hope that the healing and fulfilling work of worship will draw many? [65]

Included in this framework of the priest's liturgical life and the special relationship to the place and healing power of worship is *ritual.* In the following two chapters, more will be said about ritual as a humanizing behavior. Here we will briefly describe its place and power in the liturgy of the priest-healer.

Erik Erikson is known for his work not only in the five stages of personality development and integration, but also for his seminal study of the powerful, essential role that *ritual* plays in each stage of that development. Furthermore, he pays careful, empirical attention to the continuation of ritual as it continues to support and shape healthy adult life.

> We should, therefore, begin by postulating that behavior to be called *ritualization* in man must consist of an agreed-upon interplay between at least two persons who repeat it at meaningful intervals and in recurring contexts; and that this interplay should have adaptive value for both participants. [66]

Erikson's work in the Ontogeny of Ritualization will be used with greater specificity in the final chapters which summarize and advance my thesis that a therapeutic relationship is spiritual at its core. Here, however, I begin with a notion of ritual that suggests its symbolic ability, <u>*sui generius,*</u> to advance communion between two persons or, by extension, two *entities.* Thus we understand that rituals larger than, or outside of the context of formal, religious *worship* experiences which are occasioned by the priest-healer have a healing potential by virtue of the contextual philosophical anthropology we have presented earlier. Macquarrie frames that stance in yet another way, saying:

Tillich once wrote: *He who is not able to perceive something ultimate, something infinitely significant, is not a man.* This may seem to be just as dogmatic and sweeping an assertion as that of the secularist who dismisses God and the worship of God as relics of a past era of human experience. Are we then simply faced with two assertions? I think we must notice that there is a difference. Tillich has a richer and fuller concept of humanity than those he castigates, for he wishes to include a dimension of experience which stretches man to a new stature, while the secularists deny that there is such a dimension and impose narrower limits on what it means to be human. But man, as the self-transcending being, refuses to be arrested at the stage of a truncated nature. If he is deprived of the religious dimensions, then he is living as something less than a man in the fullest sense. [67]

We note here again that *religion* and religious ideation/formalization is understood to be part of humankind's search for meaning; and that the search itself may or may not include participation in the formalized expressions of a conscious relationship to the sacred which characterize *religions. Spirituality* will be the focus for the next chapter. We will describe its overarching hunger as one that includes religious expression. Jung ended his 1933 reflection *Modern Man in Search of a Soul* with these remarks.

The living Spirit grows and even outgrows its earlier forms of expression; it freely chooses the men in whom it lives and who proclaim it. This living spirit is eternally renewed and pursues its goal in manifold and inconceivable ways throughout the history of mankind. Measured against it, the names and forms which men have given it mean little enough; they are one the changing leaves and blossoms on the stem of the eternal tree. [68]

The *liturgy*, or work, of the priest-healer has the potential to engage the seeker whether there is a predisposition to the presence of the sacred in all of human life or not. As familiar, available and one of the chosen mediums to advance a sense of *communion* with the sacred and a larger community, both worship and ritual expression have long exhibited the potential to draw its participants into a level of mystery known to add a sense of wholeness and peace to human experience. When such a *religious attitude*, so defined as including or separate from formal religions and basic to both, is engaged, the potential for healing as the result of a fuller humanity and sense of self is awakened.

The priest-healer effects this invitation to a fuller experience of life anytime he interrupts ordinary, sleep-like, unreflective life with a moment of deeper awareness that is often sparked by symbolic activity latent with more expansive meanings. In some settings these moments occur communally during hour-long [or more] rituals of worship, formal and informal. In others, the minister, priest, rabbi or shaman may calm a person's cluttered mind with a ritual prayer, blessing or incantation. In the sacred *space* created there can follow such priestly healing as might come through silent meditation, the guidance of spiritual direction, a confessional moment of outpouring darkness and pain, an anointing to remind the sick of the presence of the sacred even in times of loss or impending death or the right-sizing of a perceived personal crisis by attending to past experiences of survival and *grace*.

Whether such moments are formalized in high church traditions and known as *sacraments*, or occur in iconoclastic religious traditions whose appeal favors *sola scriptura* and the community gathered to listen to a life-giving gospel of *good news*, the seeker is invited by the priest-healer out of his isolation and into community. Most often, and even in religious practice where explicit rituals and symbols are scarce, both individuals and communities invited to a posture of worship do so in an atmosphere marked by *prayer.*

By any definition or practice, prayer is a method of self-transcendence to a deeper reality. Whether alone or with others, when in a Christian context or a shamanic encounter, prayer can be healing.

> Prayer is not only passionate thinking, it is *compassionate* thinking. In prayer, we go out from ourselves, we stand alongside the other, we try to share feelings and aspirations. In Buddhist spirituality, there is a meditative practice known as the *Brahma-Vihara*, an expression which could quite properly be translated as *dwelling with reality.* Prayer is not, as is sometimes alleged, a flight or an escape from reality. It is a dwelling with reality in the sense of a compassionate confrontation in thought with human beings in their actual situations. [69]

As the priest-healer is an acknowledged, informed, prepared person of faith in a world whose bounds are not contained by the material or the visible, his invitation to either communal or individual prayer grounds the seeker in a humanity whose humanness is more complete by reason of communion with a reality imbued with the spiritual.

Part III -- A word about Efficacy

Those healers who have been gathered under the aegis of *priest* stand on already sacred ground. Their very existence in the community announces a basic orientation to human experience and meaning which allows and fosters the spiritual. The image which begins this chapter captures but one, formalized, specific ceremony known to me by memory during college and, later, through my own priestly call and ordination in the Roman Catholic tradition. With a larger lens we have included in *priest-healers* all whose very life, their *liturgy*, is a work of making known and efficacious the healing potential of communion with the sacred, the holy -- indeed, Rudolf Otto's the *wholly other*. In our operative framework, those called to positions of priestly service – whether formally ordained in religious services or called by their own heroic passage of suffering-made-healing – have had their conscious awareness transformed by both belief and experience.

Believing in the numinous, and having encountered the wholeness offered, priestly healers become available in primitive and contemporary cultures to give of that which they know and have received. Their training in formal programs may have taken parallel academic and devotional tracts. In less formal settings, it may have been that of curiosity turned to discipleship. In any case, it is the sacred, Otto's *mysterium tremendum*, which has drawn them in and convicted them of what we have referred to as a *religious attitude*.

In speaking briefly of the efficacy of healing within the spiritual framework we have fashioned thus far, it is important to note that history and comparative religious studies, as well as theology, paint a very broad landscape as to how or why *priestly healers* effect such experiences of attitudinal transformation, spiritual conversion or even physical healing. That discussion is beyond our concern here except where it touches a pivotal notion we used earlier in discussing the impact of a *spiritual* or *sacred* orientation to human existence. There we used the notion of *awakening* to the presence of the holy, the sacred dimensions of experience and their power to heal. The Psalmist tells us that the rain cannot fall to the ground without having its effect [Psalm 147]. Spiritual writers across traditions claim that encountering the sacred is qualitatively distinct from greater self-consciousness. The awakening that follows holds inherent opportunities for growth into fuller personhood. I have pointed out that capacity for transcendence resides in us *qua* human, and that transcending human finitude is both a reflection of a *power greater than ourselves* – a wholly other – as well as a personal *conversion* [lat. to *turn toward*] in the direction of fuller personhood. As the capacity for transcendence lies within us created *imago dei*, so does the potential for fuller personhood lie in awakening.

Groeschel speaks of the efficacy of the encounter with the numinous and frames the response, or potential for growth, as a matter of degree and choice. While I have not used the term *grace* thusfar, the reader will recognize it as one of many ways to describe the gratuitous experience of human awakening to the spiritual dimension of life itself.

> To the degree that a person responds to the awakening – for response is always necessary – life will be changed. One person may turn away and the experience of grace will pursue him – to borrow Francis Thompson's expression – as he flees 'down the nights and down the days' until he is caught. Another person may turn away and the invitation will not be extended again, as ... in the case of Bertrand Russell. Yet another will be haunted by it, as James Joyce was, never quite able to stifle the call, yet never really answering it. Still others will

respond totally like St. Francis. On the basis of a single experience at San Damiano, Thomas of Celano could say that Francis had become a different man. [70]

There have also been, and remain, places in theological discourse where the distinctions between magic and ministry are blurred. Thusfar we have positioned the priestly healer as a kind of bridge-builder, a kind of John The Baptist [in the Christian Tradition] who points the way toward moments and sources of spiritual conversion or awakening. Yet some understandings of spiritual efficacy and healing locate efficacious power solely in the healer. Generally speaking, and only by way of elucidating our contrary position here, these theological constructs seem attached to ontological changes in the *priest* as conferred upon that person either by religious ceremony or his own passage through a transforming period of life. This view of efficacy suggests that by virtue of the priest's call and the *powers* granted him, the power to change or effect healing reside within the priest, and exert influence when rightly performed [e.g., *ex opere operato*]. Although not the only example in the history of religion, certainly the reformation debate about priestly status, power and authority within the Christian church finds its own expression, inclusive of debate, even to this day.

The efficacy resident in the priestly healer I speak of in this thesis would support the transformative power of the healer's journey into suffering followed by a return to fuller personhood and a vocation of guiding others along its path. In this sense, power does reside in the priest. It is power that born of a spiritual awakening, conviction and a sense of mission. The attitude is generically *religious* as we have described it. The conviction is grounded in a philosophical anthropology that admits of more than can be framed in *secular* stances toward the world and life itself. Mission or vocation comes from both formal and informal training periods and the recognitions of a priestly role within the community which accompany these.

In presenting a spiritually grounded and trained healer [priest], we have proposed a person associated in some recognized fashion as given to the potential for human wholeness which is born of communion with the *sacer*, the holy.

Efficacy, therefore, is a function of consciously and intentionally drawing another, or a whole community, into a greater awareness of life in its sacred fullness. As Goeschel reminds us, ...*the awakening of one person may radically affect the lives of others, as with the founders of religious institutes, ... Another person answering it may be so private as to be known only after death. An example of the latter type is Dad Hammarskjold whose reminiscences in diary form were never intended for publication.*[71] Such fullness may be further described, even dogmatized, through theological conceptualizations which unfold in those traditions over time. The healer-priest, in our more generic framework, is one who – by any route or identification – stands within a tradition informed by the spiritual and invites seekers to a new level of consciousness which gives the presumed spiritual hungers of humankind nurture. *Despite the particular circumstances, one fact is certain: When the awakening occurs in a person of real depth and dimension, and it is accepted or rejected, the person will never be the same again.* [72]

The work of this chapter will be augmented in those which follow. A critical place in the whole of this thesis, however, belongs to the efficacy of myth and ritual so natural to the priest as healer. As we have given myth a place in our discussion already, I end this section with the words of Nagandra, and an emphasis on the unitive, healing power of ritual.

Considered as a continuous series of actions oriented to an end, life is an incomplete process, its true essence lies in its relation to the whole which it constantly tries to express. Ritual from this point of view may be regarded as an expression of its primordial existential urge for integration with the whole that transcends and transfigures it. [73]

Chapter Three Notes

[57] Vatican Council II Documents, op. cit., pg. 881
[58] Vatican Council II Documents, op. cit., pg. 894
[59] Morgan, *Scholar, Priest and Pastor*, op. cit., pg. 7
[60] ibid., pg. 16
[61] Crowley, op. cit., pg. 15
[62] Otto, op. cit., *The Idea of the Holy*, pg. 6-8
[63] Macquarrie, op. cit., *Paths In Spirituality*, pg. 17-18
[64] Macquarrie, John: *Principles of Christian Theology* [1977] Charles Scribner's Sons, NY, pg. 150
[65] Macquarrie, op. cit., Paths In Spirituality, pg. 18
[66] Worgul, George S., Jr.: *From Magic to Metaphor* [1980] Paulist Press, New York, pg. 53
[67] Macquarrie, op. cit., *Paths*, pg. 22
[68] Jung, Carl G.: *Modern Man in Search of a Soul* [1933] Harvest Book/Harcourt Brace & Co., London, pg. 244
[69] Macquarrie, op. cit., *Paths*, pg. 27
[70] Groeschel, Benedict J.: *Spiritual Passages* [1992] Crossroad, NY, pg. 74
[71] ibid., pg. 75
[72] ibid.
[73] Worgul, op. cit., pg. 64

Chapter Four
The Spiritual Journey

Part I – Facing Darkness – The Path to Light

The title may sound trite, esoteric, or even tainted with *new age* jargon. So much has been written about spirituality from so many perspectives. The literature is broad and escapes simple categorization. As the post-modern search for things spiritual seems to be expanding exponentially through books, magazines, television and other such media, clearly interest in spirituality is ubiquitous. Furthermore, when the object or proper end of our human capacity for transcendence is best described as *ineffable*, the plethora of words, vantage and starting points, images employed and historical-cultural frameworks meant to capture that which eludes the confines of rational expression tend to be ever more expansive in overcoming its word-bound search. As I honor the complexity of the subject, and to focus in this chapter on a few foundational concepts pertaining to spirituality as it pertains to my thesis, I begin once again with an image that comes from my more current experience as counselor – a kind of anecdotal case study so to speak. It also begins to disclose a basic sense of the *spiritual* I have in mind.

My first full time employment, following departure from active ministry, was as Director of Community Residence Programs of a local NYS Certified Drug and Alcohol Treatment Agency. Among other management, leadership and staff supervision responsibilities, I had the responsibility of developing the *community residence* model of the *therapeutic community.*

Such a model is hardly the invention of the addiction recovery movement. Other mental health facilities have long used the residential setting as part of therapy. In our case, recovery included group therapy as well as an environment meant to bring back into the life of our residents an integration of physical, emotional and spiritual wellness. Much like the apostolic church reflected in the Acts of the Apostles in the Christian tradition, this model adheres to at least four constants in the rhythm of community life: First is the message of hope [viz., salvation; *faithful to the teaching of the apostles* Acts. 2:42]. That message required a deepening of both intellectual understanding and soulful appropriation of recovery for each resident in the context of community support. This took the form of community meetings, group therapy, *activities of daily living* rehabilitative sessions [viz. prayer as earlier described, cf. Macquarrie; viz. brotherhood, Acts 2:42]. Their common life together over a period of three to six months was given form and structure by a schedule whereby they *distributed the proceeds of their goods and possessions among themselves according to what each one needed* [Acts 2:44]. As the *Big Book* of Alcoholics Anonymous indicates, there is, on a daily basis, less sharing of material possessions and more emphasis on hope by living in an atmosphere free of alcohol and drugs. Residents have multiple opportunities to be transparent about the poverty of chemical dependency and the hope of recovery. They each in turn share their *experience, strength and hope* in the context of therapy sessions, community and AA meetings, and shared leisure time. So too, this model provided for *celebrations* of progress both in daily meals and during special occasions where periods of newly attained sobriety were recognized, for example, at three months, six months etc. [cf. Acts. 2:42,46]

This analogous glance at one religious community's early life describes many current models of therapeutic, or healing, communities. Fundamental in both the AA literature and the early Christian community is the admonition to a diaconal expression in service, or, euphemistically, *giving back* to the community even beyond its borders. In the AA model, such service work occurs in both the sharing of one's story [recovery/salvation] as a kind of testimony, as well as the more explicit charge to keep one's sober living by attending AA meetings and reaching out to the *still suffering alcoholic* through prayer, support, sponsorship and actual interventions. *Having had a spiritual awakening as a result of these steps, we tried to carry this message to alcoholics, and practice these principles in all our affairs.* [cf. Alcoholics Anonymous, *How it Works*, Step Twelve.]

Acknowledging that this is not a thesis given to establishing the spiritual validity of the AA program, the image is sufficiently useful in beginning a discussion of spirituality to stay with the example for a moment. Therefore, the question comes: What Steps; what principles are to be *applied in all our affairs?*

Millions of people all over the globe have found the AA program critical in moving from the slavery of addiction to the freedom of embracing a spiritually based life. Alcoholics Anonymous is not at all shy about its spiritual orientation. *Our personal adventures before and after [entrance into the program; recovery] make clear three pertinent ideas:*[cf. *Big Book* of AA, How It Works, pg. 60]

a)   That we were alcoholic and could not manage our own lives.

b)   That probably no human power could have relieved our alcoholism.

c)   That God could and would if He were sought.

Of particular note in the Twelve Steps of AA relative to its explicit, however general, spiritual foundations are steps Two, Three and Eleven: [cf. *Big Book* of AA, pg. *59*]

> Step Two: Came to believe that a Power greater than ourselves could restore us to sanity.
>
> Step Three: Made a decision to turn our will and our lives over to the care of God *as we understood Him.*
>
> Step Eleven: Sought through prayer and meditation to improve our conscious contact with God as we understood Him, praying only for the knowledge of His will for us and the power to carry it out.

The Oxford Movement, which ultimately inspired the formation of AA, sought to translate some of the basic principles of spirituality so as to render to those both inside and outside of formal religious bodies a schema applicable to any seeker. In its practical wisdom, AA has built what many judge to be a successful organization whose traditions labor hard to keep it far removed from either a religion or a cult. Stated at every meeting as part of the AA traditions, *There are no dues or fees for membership; our leaders are but trusted servants, they do not govern; AA has no opinion on outside issues, lest problems of money, property or prestige divert us from our primary interest; the only requirement for membership is a desire to stop drinking... .* [The Twelve Traditions of AA]

The insights and foundational assumptions evident in the Oxford Movement's discourse which seem to translate most simply and clearly to spiritually-based programs like AA are seen as a distillation of the more complex, multifaceted story of spirituality and the spiritual journey.

What seemed to become fundamental in the recovery movement reflects some of the conceptual distinctions inherent in both an understanding of, and a search for, a spiritual life.

There is a process of being humbled by the uncontrollable events of life. Humility appropriated to a growing, health-seeking person in no way replicates the destructive traumas that may have contributed to a loss of self; it rather *redeems* it by a more balanced relationship to self, others and the cosmos – including God as understood by each of us. Joining others in the search for a more spiritual way of living is to move from isolation born of defeat and into a community seeking wholeness. Far from an abject sense of self which devalues personal gifts, talents and resources, the spiritual *surrender to a power greater than oneself* is seen as a healthy advance to seeking and utilizing *all* healing and help available in both the horizontal and vertical dimensions.

The process of recovery is to be life-long. Just as many paradigms of spiritual growth honor powerful religious/spiritual moments of *conversion*, the course of the journey is firmly set on a life of deepening one's relationship with *the holy* over time. Such a perspective also allows that the results, when they should come, of any conversion and subsequent new life will develop slowly as insight supports new behavior, and as new behavior confirms insight.

My years of ministry, preceded by theological and spiritual studies, made the transition to Director of a Community Residence seem like a natural shift. *Hope* is a theological virture as well a key element in the healing environment. The *Good News* of freedom from the slavery to addiction opened residents to another, healthier, more spiritual way of living. Sharing a common life together which required residents to share the story of their *journey out of darkness* deepened their faith in a Higher Power as well as in their own human dignity. I doubt we ever uttered the word *transcend,* but their life together offered the possibility of moving beyond suffering. In the language of AA, the program offered the chance to slowly attain gifts *beyond their wildest dreams.* Times of *celebration* were directly connected with residents' recovery process. Salvation, in this model and in many spiritual frameworks, is not a static moment of change. Community celebrations were therapeutic gatherings to recognize and become more deeply aware of another basic AA belief: *God is doing for me what I can't do for myself.* [cf. *The Promises of AA*]. These four constants in community life paralleled the on-going healing *rituals* of AA attendance, community meetings, individual and group therapy and household chores. Responsibility for maintenance of personal space, preparing meals and welcoming prospective new residents were all consciously connected to the AA program's belief in service to others. Although community life was never perfect, and community conflict often required community resolution, the structural basics of our program held up for residents both an ideal and a path to follow. At its base was an ever present spiritual foundation.

Part II – Hope and Transcendence

Because any approach to spirituality encompasses such a range of philosophical, historical, cultural and theological perspectives, I use theologian and spiritual writer John Macquarie's work to guide us through the remainder of this chapter. As foundational philosophical anthropological framework, I will turn again to the work of Rudolf Otto. A few additional authors' insights will be used to inform and widen these two pivotal sources.

In Anna Karenina, Tolstoy paints the existential stage on which the human predicament is played out.

> What I want to define is this finitude from which man cannot escape, and which his intellect must recognize as actually existent; that limitation which in fact reveals the true nature of man. I mean the inevitability of death, of struggle, of suffering and of history. For it is here, where man arrives at the ultimate limits of his sovereignty that he really begins to recognize what he really is, his actual existence. [74]

Humans are humbled by our limitations and by our suffering, and certainly by our finite status during a limited tenure on this earth. Earlier I pointed out that in such painful awareness we become *seekers* of help, i.e., therapy. Such seeking finds us approaching healers trained and prepared to assist us within the context of a relationship which we judge, and hope, will be restorative of our human potential.

While our propensity to rationality and organization of reality may separate out categories of human experience as well as professions focused on certain aspects of being human, the example of addiction used above can assist in a starting point here where a *presenting problem* masks a malady that progressively unfolds first as spiritual, then as emotional and, finally, as physical. Loss of control over one's use of a drug has been established by medical and addiction specialists as an *illness*, but one whose etiology begins with a spiritual malady, moves toward emotional chaos and finally renders a suffering alcoholic physically disabled. I find it interesting, and of no little consequence to our thesis, that *recovery* from this multi-faceted *illness* takes place in the reverse order: One begins with abstinence from the demon ravaging the body; one joins a recovery setting where relationships and support enter in; and, eventually, one begins to discover the healing help available from *a power greater than oneself.* While the illness progresses from the spiritual to the emotional and then to the physical, recovery takes hold as physical strength returns, emotional balance takes hold and, finally, as one seeks a spiritual life and continues to deepen its meaning and application for the rest of life and *in all of our affairs.*

We have presumed throughout our work the validity of approaching the appropriate professional who is best able and prepared to assist the troubled seeker according to the insight of both parties to the relationship about what the source of the problem might be. Healers of the psyche bring the valuable contributions of psychotherapy and counseling to a counselor-client relationship just as spiritual guides encourage a conscious contact with a power greater than oneself.

The intentionally reductionistic language of groups similar to AA hope to appeal to a wide sweep of troubled and ill persons whether inclined to believe in a religious dimension of life or not. There is, in fact, a section in the *Big Book of AA* known as *The Chapter to the Agnostic;* it is qualitatively reflective and invitational only. The AA program believes in a public relations policy that is captured by words read at every AA meeting: *attraction, rather than promotion.* I applaud the wisdom of such a conscious approach to naming their spiritual foundations alongside the *Steps* to recovery which their members have found experientially useful. I will discuss the priestly dimensions of healing to all therapeutic work. The work of this chapter on Spirituality and the Spiritual Journey requires a modest movement beyond such helpful, basic applications of spirituality as evidenced in AA and other such programs. Logic alone would suggest that the seeking and the receiving of help from God, a Higher Power, the sacred or even a benevolent cosmos presumes not only the very existence of such spiritual help, but humankind's potential for any manner or expression of what these programs refer to as *conscious contact* with *it.*

We come now to a brief discussion of the mediator/atrix of any spiritual contact, help, wisdom or other resultant *more* available in, and as part of, human experience. Admittedly, my approach is framed in generic language meant to keep us from complex theological speculation [theodicy] often known to result in one religion being *truer* than another. In my experience as a therapist, I often have seen communion with the holy [One] as constellated in humanity and known in human experience as an invaluable therapeutic experience. Macquarrie will again inform our theological anthropological stance; Otto will elucidate for us the qualitative, engaging element of *fascination* inherent in mystery [*mysterium tremendum*].

John Macquarrie, in his chapter on *Spirit and Spirituality*,[75] begins by noting the broad use of the word spirituality. He then connects the suspicions of some regarding religious practice to the broader collective of spirituality and wonders aloud about distinctions between them as well as whether interest might grow in one or the other – or both. History will tell the story more fully, but there is little doubt that post-modern culture is fascinated with spiritual paths and the human potential for a more complete life through accessing presupposed spiritual sources in our experience. Why would it not be so if his definition, which I embrace, is accurate?

Speaking of the several aspects of spiritual development, Macquarrie writes:

> To some it suggests a kind of hot-house atmosphere in which people are unduly pre-occupied with their own inward condition. To others it suggests a pale ghostly semi-existence in which the spiritual is contrasted with the bodily and material. To others again, the word has connotations of unctuousness and pseudo-piety. Yet, in spite of all misunderstandings, the word *spirituality* still has a certain fascination and it has been rediscovered ... This is because it points to something that is so important that no amount of distortion and perversion can ever quite destroy it. I believe that fundamentally spirituality has to do with becoming a person in the fullest sense... [76]

One has the sense that both the essence of spirituality as well as the interest in exploring its meaning are both irrepressible. Not only do I concur with that judgement, I believe contemporary experience over the last three decades demonstrates a resurgence of interest in things spiritual. However one understands the current phenomenon, a similar position is described by Miller who is a psychologist.

> For as long as people have been able to record their thoughts, they have conceived of reality in a way that is not limited to sensory experience and intellectual knowledge. Most generations and cultures have taken for granted that *this is not all there is*, that there is a spiritual dimension of reality

94

and of human nature beyond this material world we know through our senses. To be sure, the degree of emphasis on spirituality varies in pendulum fashion over the years. At the moment, in American culture at least, we seem to be coming out of a period of extreme materialism, experiencing anew the hunger for that which is transcendent in and beyond us. There are many ways to understand and experience that transcendence. Some call it by the name *spiritual,* and others do not. Some seek it through the historical avenues of religion. Some worship a deity or higher power; others find ultimate meaning in commitment to certain values or in creating gifts that will outlive them. [77]

Once familiar with both authors quoted above through a careful reading of the works containing each quote, I believe it is fair to say that both scholars imply that this is more than a recurring curiosity in a chance common interest. The theologian is clear here about his position: *spirituality has to do with becoming a person in the fullest sense;* the psychologist says as much by placing the search squarely in the human seeker: *experiencing anew the hunger for that which is transcendent in and beyond us.*

Discourse and debate about whether God created humankind or we created God is well known to most. We need not work here to establish something so well recorded. We know, too, of those who have even supplied good reasons why humans should need to find at least a conceptual way out of the mess of finitude to which we referred at the beginning of this chapter.

Yet here I take the view that may also be held based on religious faith and argued in light of the *revealed truth* proper to such a religious tradition. My view recognizes that possible directional development toward greater specificity within the world's religions; yet it neither presumes nor requires it. I approach the hungers affirmed in faith as the same hungers so often evident in humankind generally. Such hungers may not have knowledge of any sacred scripture or revelation; such hope of becoming a human person in the fullest sense may never have encountered that thought in any religious teaching. I propose this is a desire to find a religious perspective which I judge as at least *naturally available* to humankind. Whether framed in a common *hunger* for the transcendent, or a desire, however conscious, to come to full stature as a person, this pervasive human longing can be regarded as a qualitative distinction constellated within us as human. Others, like my esteemed ordinarius, may choose to simply call this a basic drive.

Remembering that we have earlier identified *religious man* more as a person whose disposition remains open to the metaphysical, and not simply as a person of an identified, formal faith tradition, I see this *naturally available* disposition asking what it means to be human. Paradoxically, the question itself is an indication of our human capacity for transcendence even as it leads to the *wholly other* in whose image we are made. Specific religions, I believe, demonstrate that religious man is a spiritual seeker primarily. Religious traditions attempt to gather and contain that which cannot be fully circumscribed with words. The importance of religious expression in the form of ritual, myth and symbol touch, in part, upon a reasonable desire to understand the ineffable – in Anselm's words, *fides quaerens intellectum.*

Together with my interest in demonstrating the spiritual dimensions of any therapeutic relationship, I take note of current interdisciplinary and interreligious dialogue for another reason. While I consider it appropriate – indeed healthy – for a person to adopt and stand within a particular religious expression as a way to anchor ones spiritual search and find community, faith grounded in the human hunger for an ineffable God is less likely to become a place in which to isolate. Our world is even now experiencing the destructive potential of rigid fundamentalism. Former Benedictine monk Bede Griffiths is one among many spiritual guides and scholars who would encourage both a religious home, or community, alongside a deep appreciation of all spiritual paths taken to a common sense of the holy. In his book, *A New Vision of Reality*, he writes:

> ... we turn to the spiritual order and the place of religion. This involves a return to the perennial philosophy, the ancient wisdom which underlies all religion from the earliest times. It will involve a respect for the traditional wisdom of primitive people, ... More and more today we are discovering the wisdom of these people, the harmony they have achieved in the lives and the very profound understanding they have of how human life is related to the natural world about them and to the world of spirits beyond them. Generally, such people evidenced an integrated, holistic view of life... we are learning, and we shall continue to learn, that all the different religious traditions, from the most primitive to the most advanced, are interrelated and interdependent, and that each has its own particular insights. For the Semitic religions in particular, Judaism, Christianity and Islam, it is important that they give up the exclusive claims which characterize them. This would free them to recognize the action of God in all humanity from the beginning of history. [78]

Robley Whitson ponders the spiritual impact if religions would give up what I interpret as a *revelational ethnocentrism*. Making an argument captured by the title of his book, *The Coming Convergence of World Religions,* Whitson examines several of the traps lurking within developed theological perspectives which, as yet it seems, necessarily end up standing in judgment over the *less true* revealed truth of other sacred sources. He seems to hope for more humility within each religious framework about the value of what is held sacred for each without de-valuing other such sacredly held and *inspired* sources.

> Putting aside the particular questions of inspiration, inerrancy and the like, and also putting aside the judgments each Tradition makes about the revelational condition of the others' books, the identification of a revelational situation with the production and preservation of sacred writings should create at least theological embarrassment upon noting that *non revelational* Traditions also have books regarded as sacred and as essentially linked to the shared experience. [79]

My approach to spirituality is located first in the *experience* of being human, and only after that in the constructs and conceptualizations as rational thought might conspire to express it. This is in no way misses or minimizes the important distinctions belonging to humankind by virtue of our ability to be in relationship with self, others and the cosmos. A spiritual hunger is rather at the root of that same reflective, creative human quality. Noting the several references to human *existence* and *experience* in this chapter's work thus far, I again turn to Macquarrie's cogent formulation of the religious dimension of experience as both a source of spiritual longing, and, therefore, as the naturally available compass to its nurture. In this framework, theological expression and formulations of particular religious traditions take their place as indicative of a coexisting desire and propensity for rational humankind to give shape to a felt religious response – a kind of *reflection on experience* of which is he also capable.

In the broadest sense, then, it is the experience of existing as a human being that constitutes a primary source for theology; not just explicitly religious experience, but all experience in which a religious dimension is discernable. This was implied in my remark that faith meets *what seems to be a quest in the very constitution of our human existence*. But this remark implies further that although it is only in experience that we become conscious of the quest, the roots of the quest are, in a sense, prior to experience since they belong to the very structure or form of human experience. [80]

In positing that such a religious or spiritual quest is constitutive of human existence, the origins of a spiritual hunger appear without much difficulty. This *secular man* joins his human counterpart rather than being seen as another *type*, or a departure of some sort. Macquarrie invokes theologian Langdon Gilkey who argues *that elements of what he calls 'ultimacy' and 'sacrality' are present in secular experience.*

Acknowledging that for the secular man an explicitly religious experience of the ultimate is lacking, he claims that 'ultimacy' has not thereby vanished – and could not vanish – from modern experience; on the contrary, it is present, as it has always been in human life, as a base, ground and limit of what we are, and presupposition for ourselves, our thinking, our deciding and our acting. [81]

Macquarrie concludes that ...*The quest of which have spoken is then present in experience from the beginning. In the broadest sense it is a quest for self-understanding and it has theological significance to the extent that it comes to grips with the religious dimensions of experience.* [82]

Otto's work sheds the brightest and broadest light on what I have been calling the religious dimensions of experience. The bridge from *rational analysis* to a sense of the numinous is religious in character. It is a response elicited by an encounter with the spiritual dimension of life and its very author, the wholly other. Communion with the sacred is not only naturally available to religious man, but it is also an invitation to fuller personhood [cf. Macquarrie] and, therefore, healing.

The notion of spiritual hunger being *awakened* in us by a variety of life experiences is commonplace in the journals of spiritual direction. While such writings may take a certain type of religious, even denominational, stance, such an awakening suggests a response to something, or someone, that is – in Otto's language – *wholly other.* Otto himself has wrestled with the rational components of religious ideation and encourages others to do likewise. Yet after that effort, he cautions us to carefully weigh the contrast between rationalism and profounder religion. Avoiding the *human nature* debates, I find Otto's work provides for me the basis for making distinctions between the content of religious ideation and all spiritual stirrings inherent in human experience. Otto's theological anthropology sheds light by providing the _fundamentum in re_ of religious experience.

Rather than moving from a framework of what is *natural* in human nature, and what is not, Otto avoids what I think of as a philosophical escape clause necessarily invoked once one reality is judged *natural* and another not. He notes and then moves beyond the notion of *un- or supra-natural* whose validly becomes of consequence once such a construct of humanity is assumed. Stating that *It is not that which is commonly asserted, that rationalism is the denial, and its opposite the affirmation of the miraculous. ... For the traditional theory of the miraculous as the occasional breach in the causal nexus in nature by a Being who himself instituted and therefore must be master of it – this theory is itself as massively 'rational' as it is possible to be.* [83] *The difference between rationalism and its opposite is to be found elsewhere. It resolves itself rather into a peculiar difference of quality in the mental attitude and emotional context of the religious life itself.*[84]

I do not suggest that Macquarrie and Otto are joined in any carefully crafted or tightly conceptualized approach to things spiritual. What I do find helpful and complimentary in their work is both foundational and intentionally generic for the work of this chapter. If there is to be a potential source for healing, indeed becoming more human, and if that spriritual source – named or not – may be present, how are we to know it?

Part III – God As Present – Named or Not

Even those of us who do not typically read instructions when putting something together usually believe at the start that we not only can do the task unaided, but that there is a kind of natural fit lurking among the scattered pieces. While both parts of that statement may be true, moments of being stuck, lost, tired or confused about just how the puzzle goes together can be catalysts for an appeal to the guidance of the enclosed instructions. We might even see these pictures and charts as kind of map pointing the way. With or without the image and printed details, the pieces have the potential of coming together and fitting properly. The instructions, if you will, mediate possibility; yet it cannot be said that they alone either cause or allow it. Potential for the communion of the whole can be said to lay – perhaps hidden or veiled – in the experience of successful joining of parts already crafted to be potentially in communion with one another.

My analogy contains an acknowledged weakness even as it tries to shed some light on the availability of the *sacer* or the *wholly other* to humanity. I use it only to suggest an image which I will try to clarify using Otto's notion of the element of *fascination* in *mysterium.* The truth of the matter is that my image calls to mind a household project or a kind of puzzle that we labor to put together by joining its various parts correctly. I mean only to suggest by it that the joining is facilitated by the map or the instructions.

Those instructions make explicit what lies implicit in the various pieces as they figuratively hunger to find the fit that will make the object to be what we sense we want and need in the first place – the completed project or puzzle. It is effectively brought together out of our desire to appropriate to our good and helpful use the object [project, goal, pleasure of puzzle-completion] that had drawn our interest or fascination in the first place. The analogy admittedly falls short of any useful treatment of the puzzle-project's pieces being of radically different kinds or entities. Here again we have avoided the notion of the separate, similar and yet unequal aspects of various theological constructs as they speak of the nature of God and the nature of humankind.

Yet I have implied in this image what is also not being suggested, viz., the instructions or map do not *cause* there to be a coming together of the parts into a whole. Maps, charts, instructions, persons pointing the way out of their own lived experience to another who is more lost, weak, less aware and yet still wanting the parts to come together, if you will, are mediators of a communion or completion – a fullness – that lies already possible in the scattered pieces. Such a facilitating, intentional helpmate -- whether a chart of instructions or spiritually awake guide – mediates possibilities laden with hope of completion and fullness.

Many are familiar with the caricature from outside the Roman Catholic Church of its once emphasized understanding of how and why the elements of bread and wine *became* the *sacramental* presence of Christ during the *Mass*. Basically, the validly ordained priest rightly *saying the words of consecration* over the correctly constituted *elements* before him *transubstantiated* them. Little wonder, at least in hindsight, that the Latin words of consecration, *Hoc est enim corpus meum*, were critically judged by those less enamored of such a theology of priesthood as so much *Hocus pokus*.

Some forms of priestly mediators in matters religious and spiritual have been cast, or cast themselves, as the *sine qua non* of bridging the holy gap between creature and creator, profane and sacred, a sinful state and holiness, etc. In such paradigms of mediation through a *holy, Gnostic, magical or otherwise necessary mediator* [often a priest as the etymology suggests], attention goes to mechanisms of mediation – including the priestly person – rather than to the full content and capacity of human experience as we have understood it in these pages.

Regarding the notion and name of numen/numinous, Otto wished to identify and work with the *'extra' in the meaning of 'holy'...and beyond the meaning of goodness;* we have seen his intent in describing the uniqueness of this *X. (It) cannot, strictly speaking, be taught, it can only be evoked, awakened in the mind; as everything that comes 'of the spirit' must be awakened.* [85] Otto eventually departs from Schleiermacher by essentially locating the experience of the *numen* as something of a response that is *praesens,* present, as it was for Abraham. Its awareness-referent exists outside the self and is not merely sensed in a peak moment of dependence or simple self-consciousness.

Here is Otto's *wholly other,* which is not merely a self-reflective moment of awareness whose only referent is oneself. Daunting yet approachable, Otto's *mysterium tremendum is for him not merely something to be 'wondered' at but something that entrances him; and beside that in it which bewilders and confounds, he feels a something that captivates and transports him...* [86]

Otto's *Idea of the Holy* moves from distinctions he judges particular to an encounter with mystery, to the naming of it as a qualitative power whose referent is outside the self. Thus he judges, as I understand him through inference, that the feeling awakened in humankind by the *numinous* is, at very minimum, causally connected with the very source of the response which is awakened in us: The *wholly other.* At first glance, I believe it possible to understand Otto as focusing on a kind of esoteric call from that *Other* to humankind's capacity for mysticism. However, while talk of rapture and losing oneself in nothingness – a positive experience as he describes it – can be identified most obviously in moments or movements of overwhelming power, I believe he finally leads us to a *religious dimension of experience* similar to that spoken of by Macquarrie.

> On the one hand the 'magical' identification of the self with the *numen* proceeds by means of various transactions, at once magical and devotional in character – by formula, ordination, adjuration, consecration, exorcism & etc.; on the other hand are the *shamanistic* ways of procedure, possession, indwelling, self-fulfillment in exaultation and ecstacy. All these have, indeed their starting point in magic, and their intention at first was certainly simply to appropriate the prodigious force of the numen for the natural ends of man. But the process does not rest there. Possession of and by the numen becomes an end in itself; it begins to be sought for its own sake... methods of asceticism are put into practice to attain it. In a word, the *vita religiosa* begins. [87]

As I try to understand and capture the progression of Otto's thought, I find myself recalling theorists of early childhood development making the case for the normative experience during early human life of magical thinking. Such periods of adaptive thinking will later be tested by harsher realities of life. Hopefully, emotional growth will provide ways of handling such realities. Yet that is not to say that the same kind of fascination with the practical or possible does not negate an appeal to magic. The beginnings of the *vita religiosa* may come to us in mere curiosity, intriguing possibilities or engaging fascination with what lies in and before us as humans seeking the *more*, our potential.

Potential can be cast as projection. More than a few have judged the future to be an illusion, and our finitude simply that. In approaching the spiritual journey, we do well, I believe, to consider again the theological insights of theologian John Macquarrie and the work of the religious philosopher Rudolf Otto.

> ... this notion of *transcendence* better expresses the dynamic character of man's being – it is his very nature to be always transcending or passing beyond any given stage of his condition. Also the traditional word *spirit* expressed something of the same idea, for it was the endowment with spirit that allowed man to be creative and responsible and to rise above the lower levels of life. But whether we speak of existence, transcendence, or spirit, we have in mind humanity as an unfinished, open kind of being, moving into possibilities that have still to be unfolded. [88]

To return for a moment to the example which began this chapter, it is the suffering person whose pain and plight might lead him by some route to a therapist, agency or, perhaps, a trusted friend. Surviving life's experiences resides in both persons as well as in the nexus of their meeting. Long before recovery begins, some human insight or awareness enters experience suggesting that one need not feel hopeless. In this example, a friend holding out an option containing the seeds of hope, a place to begin a search, may be exercising a healing role, even mediating an opportunity. Illness, recovery and the bridge itself resides in the human experience underlying all three. I mean simply to characterize the appeal that wellness has when one is sick. Extending the image a bit, better management of one's life is often prized when things seem chaotic. Companionship might be sought during times of loneliness. The possibility of a better life may be imagined despite one's feeling adrift and lost in a sea of problems.

Len Sperry, psychiatrist and spiritual writer, observes that *the spiritual domain includes all religious and spiritual experiences, feelings, thought and beliefs about one's relationship to God and all that may transcend one's self.* [89] I have tried to establish in this chapter that a statement like this presupposes not only *being human*, but human *experience* itself is the normative, qualitative distinction in being human. It begins in the capacity for self-reflective activity, and moves beyond the self in a transcendental way of being. The natural constellation of human openness to *more* includes the capacity to encounter and navigate relationships not only with others forming culture, community, society and the like. This capacity hungers for the kind of fullness of being human, including meeting, being engaged by and deepening a relationship with the sacred, spiritual, *holy dimensions* of human experience.

Although I have intentionally left to theological speculation and specific religious understandings the names, attributes and anthropomorphic conceptions of a deity, I agree with Otto, *et. al.*, that the referent of the *numinous* is not a mere projection of either fear or awe. Rather, this *wholly other* exists beyond the self and engages us as humans ever seeking our potential. This Holy One draws us into a fascination with life at its very source. So too, it is precisely a life marked with finitude, with polarities of anxiety and hope, both of which frame our hunger for transcendence, the sacer, and invites both therapist and the troubled to draw from its well.

Chapter Four Notes

[74] Frank, Eric: *Philosophical Understanding and Religious Truth* [1994] New York/Oxford University Press, pg. 6
[75] Macquarrie, op. cit., *Paths*, pg. 40
[76] Ibid.
[77] Miller, op. cit., pg. xvii

[78] Griffiths, Bede: *A New Vison of Reality* [1989] Templegate Publishers, Springfield, Illinos, pg. 287

[79] Whitson, Robley Edward: *The Coming Convergence of World Religions* [1992] The United Institute; The Cloverdale Library, Bristol, Indiana, pg. 149

[80] Macquarrie, op. cit., *Principles*, pg. 6

[81] Ibid, pg. 7

[82] Ibid.

[83] Otto, op. cit., *The Idea*, pg. 3

[84] Ibid.

[85] Ibid., pg. 6

[86] Ibid., pg. 31

[87] Ibid., pg. 33

[88] Macquarrie, op. cit., Principles, pg. 62

[89] Sperry, Len: *Transforming Self and Community* [2002] The Liturgical Press Collegeville, Minnesota, pg. 57

Chapter Five
Therapist as Priest

Virtually anyone with small children, or grandchildren, is aware of Disney's *The Lion King*. Perhaps some have even seen its stage format. Not only do I appreciate the myth, symbol and ritual that unfolds in the movie version, I have actually used the video as part of a presentation concerning *healing* to literally hundreds of therapists, pastoral professionals and healthcare providers.

Images help me to frame a springboard for more focused work. I find two sections of the movie format very pertinent to my notion of therapist as priest. The first section will introduce this chapter; the second will help to conclude it.

With powerful drumbeats, chant-filled music and wonderful animation, the Lion King opens with a gathering of all who populate the kingdom. Birds change their direction of flight and prairie herds thunder across the plane toward *Pride Rock*. Smaller creatures ride larger ones like a taxi as the procession of life is drawn by a ritual call to gather for a special ceremony of dedication. King Mufasa and his mate have given birth. Young Simba is to be *dedicated. All* are to witness and join the celebration as the *Circle of Life* crescendos louder in the background. Elton John's voice sets the scene as every species in the kingdom gathers:

There's far too much to take in here. More to do than can ever be done. As the sun rises high in the crimson sky... It's the circle of life.

The first one to come before the King's presence does so from the skies. Azu is of the clown sort throughout the drama, yet he has the serious task of being the King's messenger. A faithful, feathered friend to Mufasa, he swoops from the skies, lands on the protruding rock-throne and reverentially bows to the Lion King. The king in turn bows and Azu takes his place. Immediately after the messenger's arrival, and with the community of creatures gathered in anticipation, a baboon equipped with staff and attached satchel makes his entrance. The crowd parts, and Rafiki, seeming every bit a shaman, passes through their midst.

As the deft, wide-eyed baboon climbs the rock and ascends to the throne, his entrance and reception are remarkably distinct from that of the messenger. A bow is replaced with the wide grin of acceptance and delight as both the King and the priestly presider warmly embrace each other. Perhaps it is true that the affinity between spiritual and secular *power* is as old as it is deep.

Rafiki goes about his work, his liturgy. Looking down at the young cub, he gets his attention first with a gaze, and then by shaking some sort of crude *rattle*. Simba's eyes follow. Rafiki has not only engaged the one about to be dedicated, but the whole community as well. They are fascinated, drawn in. The only people in the audience who seemed to miss the power of that simple ritual action were, I believe, the religious fundamentalists who were reported to have quickly rejected the movie as *satanic*, and therefore *dangerous*. Disney had allowed both a *shaman* and *magic* to fill the minds of children. Watching more closely, a mere healer using ritual might be seen.

Another ritual activity follows. Bits of sand are scooped from Simba's den and gently sprinkled on him. Rafiki steps back; Simba coughs and then sneezes. My memory drifted to a time in the Roman Catholic Baptismal ritual for infants

110

when salt was placed on the tongue. I remembered, too, that among some believers it was said that if the infant cried when the water was poured, the devil had escaped. Religious symbolism is polyvalent. It will always allow *superstition* even when it does not intentionally invite it. I know nothing of Disney's intent in the animated segments. I simply found myself engaged, fascinated and *open* to what might follow. Like Simba, I was being awakened to the moment in its ritualistic unfolding.

What follows is the cub's being transported by the shaman, held safe and lovingly in his arms, and then lifted high before the animal kingdom below. Wild, wonderful noises rise up while zebra kneel and elephants lift their trunks. Simba's small eyes widen as his little body is rotated east to west; all behold the future King. The skies open; light streams forth. By now the *rightly religious* would have left the theatre or turned off the VCR. They would have missed the *theophany* – rays of sunlight streamed from parted clouds and pointed to the newly dedicated King with heightened contrast.

The opening ends as dramatically as it had begun. With a loud burst of percussion, the next scene our eyes and hearts take in is focused on the one who didn't attend. He is alone in darkness. His name is *Scar* and he is quietly caught up in himself. An unsuspecting mouse has his attention. Scar, you see, is hungry.

Perhaps the Lion King is just a good story – a well animated and crafted one at that. Yet it seems to me there must always be more to a good movie, novel, play or a peoples' folk tale than simply the elements that capture our senses. When the bits and pieces of a story begin to engage our imagination and captivate it, research suggests that we are moving toward an ever more *conscious relationship* with a distinct aspect of reality. Certainly one way to understand the lure of a *good story* is to begin by appreciating whatever *mythical* aspects and elements it may contain. Few have shed more light on the power of myth than Joseph Campbell.

Reminiscent enough of the exact words of the song opening the Lion King to make me wonder if it was a direct reference, *The Circle of Life* states in multiple ways that life is so full and wondrous as to be mysterious. Its mystery is impossible to be totally fathomed. *There is far too much to take in here, ... more to see than can ever be seen.*. About myth, Campbell begins a chapter with these thoughts:

> Whether we listen with aloof amusement to the dreamlike mumbo jumbo of some red-eyed witch doctor of the Congo, or read with cultivated rapture thin translations from the sonnets of the mystic Lao-tse; now and again crack the hard nutshell of an argument of Aquinas, or catch suddenly the shining meaning of a bizarre Eskimo fairy tale: It will always be the one, shape-shifting yet marvously constant story that we find, together with a challengingly persistent suggestion of *more remaining to be experienced than will ever be known or told.* [emphasis added]. [90]

Campbell's fundamental assertion about stories evidencing mythical qualities is based on a life filled with cross-cultural research concerning the content of the great myths themselves. If there is a mythical element in the whole of the story of Simba in the Lion King, for example, it has to do in the first instance with the function of myth as we bring it to consciousness. That is to say, once we are in relationship with such a story either by turning our attention to it or having our normal behaviors and activities somehow interrupted by its power, we are drawn into an aspect of our human experience which Jung might label archetypal and which Macquarrie might see to be part of a human hunger for fullness. In any case, both, I believe, would concur with Campbell in seeing the qualitative distinction of *the mythical* in our stories, dreams and experience as it *transcends* that which is smaller, particular and personal in our individual lives and cultures. In *The Hero With A Thousand Faces* Campbell writes:

> It has always been the prime function of mythology and rite to supply the symbols that carry the human spirit forward, in counteraction to those other constant human fantasies that tend to tie it back. In fact, it may well be that the very high incidence of neuroticism among ourselves follows from the decline among us of such effective spiritual aid. [91]

The story of Simba unfolds in such a way as to provide analogous insight into, and common turf with, my client's stories of transformative and healing experiences. The similarities reside not in the particularities of time, culture or surrounding events containing the polarities of anxiety and hope. As Campbell reminds us, *The wonder is that the characteristic efficacy to touch and inspire deep creative centers dwells in the smallest nursery fairy tale...* [92]

What I see infallibly offered in the power of certain myths is the hope of transformation even in the face of finitude. Whether it be the image of a dragon in a folk tale or an impending medical diagnosis, a healthy spirituality embraces the whole of human experience as it realistically faces the causes of anxiety and the search for hope. In our work thus far we have aligned ourselves with those who see both elements, and other polarities as well, in the experience of being human. Navigating those polarities, as with all of human life, often begins in awareness of light which counterbalances deadly darkness; hope that ameliorates anxiety; universals which transcend particularity; life that transcends death.

For Campbell, as well as for many scholars of religion and spirituality [not even to mention the brilliantly simple self-help programs such as AA], symbol and ritual play a critical role in terms of an invitation or initiation into the spiritual journey of transformation. It follows, therefore, that those professed to assisting people in any healing journey, wherein navigating the polarities of human experience is consciously undertaken, stand on sacred ground. Consciously or not, such healers can see themselves as positioned at the brink of a collaborative healing process involving self, the client and the very source of transcendent potential.

As such, there can reside in healers the powerful dimension of symbol. The validly gained and communally recognized applied knowledge of their profession is far from a satchel of magic. Healers embrace life as it is. Magic seeks to change it.

For both therapists and priests, *symbol, ritual and story* become an efficacious dimension of healing as the result of spiritual growth and human transformation. Campbell raises to the level of *hero* the one who has taken the great transformative journey through necessary risk and suffering. It is a characteristic of *shamanic* healing not only to return from such life-changing journeys in order to accompany others just entering the same frightening path, but to return as needed to the *nether world* in order to attain wisdom and strength for the particular healing task at hand. *This stands to reason in a shamanic culture, where the shaman, as well as being a healer, serves as philosopher/priest who is privy to the supernatural.* [93]

Even if the therapist or priestly healer is not given, or eschews, the aura of *hero* by those who have trained, mentored, licensed or approached him for service, I suggest that as healers, both therapists and priests can be consciously seen as symbols. Healers can consciously choose to present themselves in a non-anxious manner. As professionals who are aware of their calling and the hope they extend to clients, both therapists and priests welcome clients to a safe, comfortable environment. Their dependable presence at the time of a scheduled appointment increases a client's sense of trust in their care as well as respect for them as persons who are vulnerable. Regular cycles of meeting times can establish a ritual which enhances and supports an expectation of a positive outcome. Attention to the client's agenda is yet another way in which the therapist or priest steps aside and makes emotional space for the client's needs. Symbols and rituals that constellate their professional practice contain, de facto, an enticing, engaging healing potential whose power flows both from human experience as well as its very source. *Religious man* may be quicker to name the *numen* and give descriptive titles like *God, The Divine, The Wholly Other etc.*; but it is the human experience of polarity and paradox which can awaken a response to *mysterium tremendum et fascinans* in any seeker regardless of the reason for risking the journey into a greater fullness of life itself. The *hero* has done so. So too do therapists and priests who also profess, and symbolize, a potential for healing.

Turning briefly to the example of addiction and recovery, the presentation of an illness, *dis-ease* or spiritual malady have a slow, insidious progression. Unlike the sudden introduction of trauma bringing someone to an emergency room, the disabling phase of emotional or spiritual unrest may be the *presenting face* of a process begun earlier and with less pronounced dysfunction. When life seems to hedge closer to the *anxiety* side of a polarity, help – the thought of it as well as the accompanying anxiety – might be sought. Attention is drawn from the routine activities of living by the gathering experience of suffering – whether an actual or perceived *crisis*. At such times, cognitive and sensory processing of the environment can awaken one to feel the need for help in order to change.

The perception of *crisis* – which etymologically signals *change* and does not presume trauma – engages us at several levels. Our human experience is put in relationship to an aspect of reality which interrupts, shifts or otherwise qualitatively engages our self-awareness. The condition of ordinary routine is faced with unusual sensations of anxiety, threat or even harm. *The motif of these processes is that of death and rebirth... and which can occur for each of us daily. This is the 'essence' of transformation, the necessity of sacrifice by the ego, the necessity of pain.* [94]

In the case of the chemically dependent person, who typically *reaches out or passes out* during later stages of the gripping progression, therapists, willing family members, clergy offering support and AA members alike become symbols of hope and possibility. Acceptance into a Twelve-Step program of recovery might, at first, simply provide a less destructive routine than the potentially lethal pattern of drug abuse. It is also true for many who suffer from addiction that the acceptance of some form of treatment, including the very act of approaching a healer, marks the existential *acceptance* of one's finitude, and a desire to move toward hope and freedom from addiction. Both ends of the *anxiety-hope polarity* still exist. Healing begins to happen when a horizon of hope becomes brighter than the weight of anxiety. Those extending hope do so in a variety of ways including a conscious relationship with the journeys they themselves have taken and the healing skills and symbols at their disposal. Therapists, like priests, have the option of consciously and intentionally incorporating this spiritual dimension of healing into their practice.

Becoming a member of something requiring only the desire and willingness to change puts a welcoming face on the first few phases of the classic schema in Van Gennep's *Rites of Passage.* [95] *Separation* from old behavior; a *liminal* state of *transition* wherein one is neither deathly ill nor as yet spiritually engaged; and, later, *incorporation* into a fellowship marked first by hope and later a healthier way of living. Along with a sponsor who is clearly a guide for understanding and *working the Steps*, fellow members become tangible symbols of a program that launches the neophyte on a daily journey to wellness. The *ritual* of attendance at meetings is further enhanced by the stability of the meeting format, which is essentially standard around the globe. While the only aspect of AA that approaches *dogma* is the grounded belief in the possibility of life-long recovery based on the lived experience of its members, the program's *creedal statements* contained in the Twelve Steps and Traditions -- as well as the testimony of the founders as contained in the *Big Book* -- become a ritual part of every meeting. Within the recommended formats for their gatherings, recovering members share their *experience, strength and hope* hinged directly on surrender to a *Higher Power*. As a AA participant's spiritual recovery progress deepens, many members come to name this Higher Power as *God*.

In order to begin a more specific bridge to the Therapist as Priest, I turn now to some of the explicit and implicit *contents* of the spiritual journey which seem to combine the disciplines of psychology and the practice of therapy. It is also important, I believe, to point out that religious and spiritual paths are not presumed to be, <u>de facto</u>, healthy. Therefore, a discussion of spirituality as it relates to religious sensibilities and how both relate to the therapeutic relationship is presented.

The December 2003 *Monitor on Psychology* quoted earlier contained several articles which consider the wisdom and ways of incorporating spirituality into mental health treatment. Its cover announced *Spirituality and Mental Health* with a subtitle *In practice, on campus and in research*. Both were set against a silhouetted figure seeming to be waist deep in water, hands joined and pointing toward a beautiful moonscape. In the earlier reference, I

117

drew attention to the current quest among therapy and counseling professionals to courageously acknowledge the importance of patients' spiritual longings and the various expressions given them. Here I note the cautions that were also voiced. Both seem appropriate and provide the kind of balanced approach which social scientists rightly give to theory and research.

William Hathaway, of Regent University in Virginia, acknowledges the delicacy of the matter: *Using religion as a therapeutic tool is a little controversial and still emerging.*[96] As the article continues, reference is made to the place confessional experiences have in patients whose religious past first gave them a ritual shape. The article states: *Hathaway uses spiritually guided forgiveness protocols to help clients deal with emotional problems that resulted from harm inflicted by friends or family members.* [97] Form seems to follow function. The therapist's office is not a church, synagogue, mosque or kingdom hall. Alcoholics Anonymous was decidedly careful not to create, nor compete with, places of worship. The AA *forgiveness protocol*, if you will, takes shape in fully <u>half</u> of the Twelve Steps, viz., Steps 4 – 10. In AA, the process of progressing from *insanity* through forgiveness finds its way into six of AA's Twelve Steps. This content is as appropriate a protocol for alcoholics as a different protocol would be appropriate for other problems. Forgiveness by the patient himself, by others and by God seems to play a significant role in human growth and development. Therapy is about wholeness; and wholeness is approached through healing. More significant still – however obvious – is that in these two examples both the therapist's consulting room and a self-help meeting look to pivotal understandings of spiritual growth as they inevitably surface within religious expressions. The debate seems not about whether to incorporate the insights of spirituality. The discussion in the article is essentially that of the Oxford Movement: How to do it respectfully, and in ways that neither proselytize nor seek to control. I believe it is a debate worth having as it honors the proper contribution of professionals from various fields and creates settings where clients' intellectual, emotional and spiritual integrity are consciously respected.

Dr. Carrie Doehring, a psychologist at the Iliff School of Theology in Denver, introduces a note of realism that some pastoral professionals may not welcome. *In the context of implementing these [spiritual] techniques, however, the possibility that religion may have a negative influence on a client's life – believing in an angry God, for example – should be assessed carefully so that therapy does not make emotional crises worse.* [98] Once again I welcome the balance that is framed in cautious care for the *counselor-client relationship* as a privileged place of access.

The variability among the *Monitor* articles, noted above, is revealed in the book edited by William Miller and published by the American Psychological Association, *Integrating Spirituality Into Treatment*. In Miller's work a healthy spiritual or religious openness to life's unfolding possibilities seems neither stranger nor enemy to professionals outside of specific *priestly* models of care. What might appear to some scientifically oriented healers as insight and worthy of research is to other, more spiritually conscious professionals, a statement of the obvious. Dr. Doehring is again quoted in another section of the same article:

> With religious or spiritual clients, that sensitivity and willingness to interact in a religious way helps them to trust the therapist and ... can bring a beautiful aspect of the human experience into the therapy room. Some people describe the beauty of spiritually guided therapy as experiencing a third presence in the room – a spiritual presence or God presence. There is a mystery being revealed to the

patient in that presence; it's a sort of epiphany that can be extremely useful in therapy. [99]

It has been my view in this thesis that healers whose proper professional orientation is secular or spiritual are joined by a common grounding in attributes attending classic notions of the professions. Among those which I have identified and discussed is the notion of privileged access to those seeking their help and the trust which characterizes contact with them. Prior to that is some basic feeling or understanding by the client of that which the caregiver believes – or *is professed*. In addition to degrees, licensure and the organization of the professional body itself is the place in the community held by the professional and the nature, or purpose, of the service rendered. Joining the professions together is an orientation to counselor-client relationships marked by lofty goals primarily for the common good and not one's own material advance. Marking this distinction, as we have shown, is a set of symbols and rewards that provide a large measure of the satisfaction and value attending professionals and their practice.

I again call attention to the notion of *call* or *vocation* as it seems to appear in literature about the professions. Some modest descriptions of that qualitative distinction in both the therapist-healer and the priest-healer were brought to bear in my discussion. Whether secular or spiritual in framework and orientation, the purpose of the therapist, and thus the work of the professional entering the work, seems ennobled by lofty goals of service. Like the priest, a therapist is called upon to understand his professional purpose, theoretical framework and consciously consent – or profess -- to both. In both therapist and priest, however, I intimated that beyond the power and purpose of the professional goal lay a call whose referent lies hidden within it, and perhaps beyond it. This sense of vocation shows itself in a variety of practical ways in ones practice.

Techniques proper to each may not be routinely used, nor are they always easily recognized. Yet both therapist and priest are free to consciously embrace the spiritual orientation of their profession as each works within the a particular setting for the good of the client – his full personhood.

It is critical to remember what I have often stated: Any *secular* professional may take up his work solely and solidly grounded on the goals of the profession alone. He may look entirely to the *secular city* for his definition and duties. The introduction to this thesis makes my argument plain. One can choose to understand and access a larger framework of, and a larger source within, the work of healing.

In sketching the philosophical anthropological perspective used as an operative assumption in this work, I assiduously avoided speaking of the specific faith or dogma content of individual religions. Instead, I employed the more general conceptualizations of *religious experience* and *spiritual* orientations or perspectives. While some images betrayed traditions of my own faith as I pieced them together for the sake of example, I have relied on Macquarrie's fundamental approach to *human experience* and Otto's work in conveying the *numinous* to guide any further rational analysis of the spiritual. In doing so, much of the current literature concerning spirituality can be read through those lenses without needless, and often very close-ended, debate about the *most true*. While I respect the freedom to do so, I am disinterested in anything whose primary focus is to claim superiority of one religion over another. What may appear to some as epistemological relativism is simply the desire to capture a glimpse of whom and what calls us to our potential, and how that X, as Otto puts it, might be consciously invoked by healer and client alike.

In suggesting that therapists and priests share a *vocation*, then, I am stating that, in addition to the conventional methods of treatment, something calls them to use the gifts and interests constellated in their growing *awareness of self and their 'liturgy'* for the *fully human* life of others. While priestly healers may name the name [of God, etc.] more readily and explicitly, therapist-healers seem *fascinated* by the healing power of the *numinous* as well.

Why should it not be so if the same author and source of life, however named or not, is actively approaching human experience and calling forth its potential? If the professions give room for both the rational and the mystical, and if science and religion have replaced their swords with ploughshares, cannot diversity of starting points and methods only increase the avenues leading back to their ineffable source?

Clearly, journals like the *Monitor on Psychology* hold to their social science orientation and methodology. The practitioners they represent and those who contribute to their pages give no evidence of becoming clergy, shamans or spiritual directors. The appropriate frameworks within *mental health* systems and diagnostic categories attach themselves to the goals and language of that profession. For that reason and others, our notice of psychology's interest in the *spiritual* or *religious* dimensions of human experience suggests not only the discipline's permission to do so, but also an inference regarding the proper focus of health and wholeness in both perspectives. We turn again to the *Monitor on Psychology:*

> The evidence indicates that the sense of hope, meaning and spiritual support that clients gain from discussing religious issues and drawing upon spiritual resources helps them cope better with their situation.
>
> The research is showing that spiritual dimensions brought into therapy can add something distinctive to health and well-being. ... People ask

'Is relgion just another version of a healthy social support or a positive system of meaning?' We're finding that there is something special about the religious dimension that cannot be easily reduced to traditional psychological constructs. [100]

In Psychological research into the utilization of spirituality in its healing modalities, findings that the religious dimensions add *'something distinctive' to health and well-being* and that there is *'something special about the religious dimension' that cannot be easily reduced to traditional psychological constructs* [cf. above] is not lost on the argument of this thesis. My summary and conclusions follow.

Chapter Five Notes

[90] Campbell, Joseph: *The Hero With a Thousand Faces* [1949] MJF Books, NY, pg. 3

[91] ibid., pg. 11

[92] Ibid., pg. 4

[93] Achterberg, Jeanne: *Imagery In Healing* [1985] Shambhala, Boston, pg. 19

[94] Hitchcock, John: *The Web of the Universe* [1991] Paulist Press, NY, pg. 180

[95] Van Gennep, Arnold: *The Rites of Passage* [1960] The University of Chicago Press, Chicago, pg. 11

[96] *Monitor On Psychology*, A Publication of the American Psychological Association; December 2003; Vol. 34, NO. 11: Washington, DC, pg. 40

[97] Ibid.

[98] Ibid., pg. 41

[99] Ibid.

[100] Ibid., pg. 42

Chapter Six
Summary and Conclusion

A therapist working within the framework of a secular, scientifically based profession does so with a prominent psychological and human service perspective. At no point do I suggest that the therapist be a priest in disguise. The growing interest in spirituality among these professionals may, however, give evidence of an earlier trend wherein some spiritually based scholars and practitioners have raised concerns about the *psychologization of spirituality*. To the extent that both professional orientations may have sought validation of their perspective through what some have judged as a boundary-crossing appropriation of the other's proper field of inquiry and their respective operative assumptions, current discourse – including cautious caveats – within each professional purview validate their scholarship. Since I have previously noted boundary and focus questions evident in psychological journals as their attention turned to contributions of spirituality to therapy, there is a parallel concern raised by those in the field of spiritual direction.

Len Sperry, a noted psychiatrist and spiritual writer, contends that the work of spiritual direction has both a valid tradition and a proper focus. He is also concerned that the tradition of spiritual direction not lose its inherent moral dimension, which, he judges, results in transformation of both self and the community. In *Transformation of Self and Community*, Sperry writes:

The *psychologization of spirituality* refers to the therapeutic influence that modern psychology exerts on understanding the spiritual life. Downey voices the concern that a psychologized spirituality appears *to have eclipsed the salvific as the governing category in spirituality.* The implications of such a psychologized, therapeutic, spirituality are great. Such a spirituality gives rise to *self absorption, self-preoccupation, self-fixation, even when the focus on the self is aimed at improving relationships with others. The criticism that much contemporary spirituality is mute on issues of social justice ... is not without warrant.*[101]

I welcome the cautions contained in Sperry's work as much as I find hope in journals of psychology raising concern about bringing the religious dimensions of human experience into the consulting room.

I have taken great care in this thesis to focus on the foundational aspects of humankind's potential for wholeness through appropriating to oneself the *naturally available, transcendent potential* inherent in the whole of human experience. Further qualitative distinctions which approach specific religious expression transport, in my view, the *inherent spiritual potential* captured in the philosophical framing of *religious man* to a specifically religious and theological context beyond the focus of my thesis. The combination of psychological factors and spiritual dimensions of human experience adopted by some therapists and the more recent support of this dual approach by spiritual writers form the basis of my thesis: A therapeutic relationship, fully and rightly understood, consciously referenced or not, rests on fundamental spiritual foundations. Continuing in that framework, I will highlight several experiences from my counseling and therapy activities to elucidate a few pivotal points of a secular therapeutic relationship and a spiritual orientation to healing has produced results not probable with either in isolation.

Several examples of a person becoming more consciously aware of anxiety, or a problem, have been given. Attempts to address the problem and resolve the presenting issue alone seem to fail. Help is sought. The phone call is made and a relationship between counselor and client begins as a confidential, confessional-like setting of safety is created in an atmosphere of respectful support. While relgion may invoke judgement and prescribe attention to moral imperatives early on, the later use of non- judgmental, therapeutic encounters of the analytical style clarify additional characteristics of the person who has risked trust and soulful disclosure of himself. Personal suffering and its progression to the point seeking help are manifestations of a person's early wishes for change and a more anxiety free life. Speaking as an analyst, Hillman cites two important characteristics of the therapist – *listening* and a *call to heal* as elaborated in the following quotations:

> Listening is perhaps less a problem for theologians and ministers since it is akin to meditation and prayer. Prayer has been described as an active silence in which one listens acutely for the still small voice, as if prayer were not asking and getting through to God, but becoming so composed that [He] might come through to me... Such listening, allowing the other to come through in his own way, this letting rather than trying, can lead to what is called in Jungian analysis psychic infection. This is another of the risks in an encounter. Where there is real connection and the gates open, two psyches flow together. One speaks of a *meeting of souls.* [102]

Although training and preparation of the therapist are critical in preparation for a healing profession, the *call to heal*, or the *vocational dimension*, does not come from the training alone. Neither does it reside in the skillful application of methodology as if technique is the final, and most efficacious, cause of a successful outcome in therapy. Once again, Hillman as analyst underscores the significance of the therapist's levels of self-awareness and adds the dimension of the therapist's desire to contribute to the healing. This second part of the nexus is the presence of compassionate skills.

> ... the ego for all its value as guard is not the therapist. Healing comes from our unguarded side, from where are foolish and vulnerable. This is expressed by the idea of the wounded healer, who heals through his own wounds – or needs, or call. A wound is an opening in the walls, a passage through which we may become infected and also through which we affect others. The arrows of love both wound and heal and are calls. Compassion does not flow from the ego. [103]

In psychological work, both seeker and healer wish to understand the source of suffering. For some presenting problems accurate diagnosis often indicates prescribed paths for positive change in behavior. In the case of traditional medicine, medications and other immediate therapeutic interventions are appropriately utilized. The *troubled soul* we have presumed to highlight is nonetheless still not a body attached to a mind and containing a spirit. In that light, we refer to Hillman once again in approaching a third nexus in the encounter: *The mystery of Personhood.* As we do so, I call to mind Ashley and O'Rourke's framework of *intelligent freedom* as the hallmark of personhood.

Every individual has a biography that consists in mature actualization of intelligent freedom and the manifestation of a unique personality. This life story passes through many phases of fetal and infant development before the brain can function at higher levels. Even during adult life, persons function with intelligent freedom only at certain times and in certain relations to their environment. [104]

A therapeutic encounter, indeed the whole of the therapeutic relationship, seeks to engage the *whole person.* The therapist welcomes the whole of a person, not simply the mind or psyche as a part.

Hillman's perspective on the focus of analysis follows.

Especially misleading is the notion that if we assiduously gather the details of a case we can piece together the mystery of a person. Details of life's accidents, unless they be representatively symbolic, are never essential to the soul. They form only its collective clutter and peripheral trivia and not its individual substance. The person who comes to counseling comes to be freed from the oppression with accidents, to find truth by stepping clean out of banalities which he himself recognizes as such but is obsessively trapped within. The task at this point is to leap qualitatively into the unknown, rather than to find out more by inquiring into the bits and pieces for the sake of finding a pattern. [105]

Holding to one's training and skills, a therapist can see himself, and therefore practice his profession, as a symbol of freedom able to navigate and survive safe entry in pathos. The polarities of human experience configure this eventual existential situation for humans, even though it is clearly the twists and turns of one's own experiences which might eventually rise from unconscious to conscious thoughts about his problems. As the seeker has already and at some level decided to *leap qualitatively into the unknown,* it is both the therapist and the *spiritual dimension of the therapeutic relationship* which invites entry and guides safe passage through it. I have often witnessed how a client's spirituality enhances both the clarification of his problems and opens a path to their amelioration. As I reflect on my immediate spiritual preparation for office hours with clients, I am struck by the difference in my own sense of purpose and demeanor when I take a few moments to meditate or pray for those I will soon be welcoming. Anecdotally, I remember the bishop who ordained me telling us seminarians who were going out to teach catechetics that we should *talk to God about our students as much as we talk to our students about God.*

While an intitial sense of awakening may have been caused primarily by perceived crisis or heightened anxiety, this becoming present and involved are evidence of the innate human and spiritual gifts in the seeker. Theology refers to those capacities when it speaks of our being made in the image and likeness of God [*imago dei*].

Ashley and O'Rourke continue the notion of our *more conscious* moments of freedom in this way.

> Much of the adult's life is taken up with routine – sleep, eating, relaxation – when intelligence is working at a level below that of creative freedom. Yet this same, identical person carries on the total process of living in all its phases. Getting sick and getting well are both parts of this continuous, struggling process of living development. Thus defining human personhood as *embodied intelligent freedom* presupposes a life process which goes on at many levels of activity, but which is more clearly manifest and definable by its maximum, its highest point of integration. [106]

For Hillman and analytical psychology, the nexus of *awakening* in the context of a therapeutic relationship finds resonance in both psychological and spiritual counseling. Both approaches present opportunities for healer and seeker to understand the choice to enter a healing process as more than simply a choice to talk with each other. What begins is clearly a relationship between counselor and client; yet both manifest a willingness to be in relationship with the troubling material which has urged the soul to begin a conscious search for help. Whether in a secular or spiritual setting, the journey awakens both to its story, and, in doing so, invites integration of its meaning. In Hillman's words *The right reaction to a symptom may as well be a welcoming rather than laments and demands for remedies, for the symptom is the first herald of an awakening psyche which will not tolerate any more abuse.* [107]

> Through the symptoms the psyche demands attention. Attention means attending to, tending, a certain tender care of, as well as waiting, pausing, listening. It takes a span of time and a tension of patience. Precisely what each symptom needs is time and tender care and attention. Just this same attitude is what the soul needs in order to be felt and heard. So it is often little wonder that it takes a breakdown, an actual illness, for someone to report the most extraordinary experiences of, for instance, a new sense of time, of patience and waiting, and in the language of religious experience, of coming to the center, coming to oneself, letting go and coming home. [108]

The four areas of convergence which were cited at the beginning of my summary constellate pivotal characteristics of a therapeutic relationship, namely: Listening; Compassionate Skill; The Mystery of Human

Personhood and Awakening. Each of these is also well known to students of spirituality as it is applied to a relationship with self, others and God. They also provide, therefore, a fundamental framework for healing available to both *therapist* and *priest* as we have described them throughout this work. As critical dimensions of healing they do not stand alone. Rather, each of these aspects of a therapeutic relationship invites therapists to consciously avail themselves of a merging wherein psychotherapeutic and priestly roles converge in the interest of healing. Given that goal, both therapist and priest are invited to put themselves at the service of their professions, their clients and the work of healing that has brought into being the relationship itself. As one freely and consciously enters the work therein, what may be discovered, and then honored, is not only the bits and pieces of the story, but the primal story-teller – the *wholly other.*

Therapist As Priest: The Spiritual Dimensions of a Therapeutic Relationship presents -- now both by title and discourse -- that a therapeutic relationship, fully and rightly understood, and whether consciously acknowledged or not, rests fundamentally on spiritual foundations. Healing is a privileged vocation for those who take up its mantle in any setting; the work engages both therapist and patient, priest and spiritual seeker. In conclusion, I turn now to the other segment in *The Lion King.*

Simba has grown, at least physically. His body is large and his mane full. Yet he wanders aimlessly, after having almost died in the desert sun. Not only had he witnessed the murder of his father by the trickery of Scar, Mufasa's brother, Simba believed that he was somehow complicit in his father's death – a lie perpetuated by the King's killer-brother himself. Believing himself guilty, and filled with fear and shame, Simba leaves Pride Rock and thus abdicates his rightful throne to Scar himself.

Simba is lost, at least to himself. Scar comes to power, and does so for himself. Pride Rock dissolves into the chaos of Eden after the apple.

Yet to the one who has carved Simba's name in the *book of life*, the shaman Rafiki, Simba will always be alive however hidden in the present moment. It is during an outpouring of frustration and deeply felt guilt that Simba thuds down on a log stretched across a stream. His self-stirrings and angst had been occasioned by ridicule coming from an unlikely pair of creatures – a warthog and weasel – who had earlier befriended him; but now they jeer at Simba's belief that *the stars above are the bright lives of those who had gone before him.* The truth is, his own father had told him that and Simba's recollection of it, along with the ridicule of his father's truth, jars the grown cub into passionate, soulful stirrings no longer able to be quieted by running.

Miles away, Rafiki senses Simba's coming to life again, his awakening. Joyfully exaulting *He's alive, Simba's alive,* Rafiki gathers his staff and satchel with the words, *I go to him.*

Presently there is noise in the trees above Simba's dire tree of restlessness. The unintelligible *mumbo jumbo* emanating from Rafiki's perch catches Simba's disinterested attention. Rafiki throws something into the water below the lion and the viewer sees the despondent Simba's reflection changed in a ripple of the water.

Like Yahweh *walking in the garden in the cool of the day* in Genesis, Rafiki slowly approaches Simba. The silly chant gets louder and the lion is more annoyed. *What's all that supposed to mean,* asks Simba. *It means you're a Baboon, and I'm not,* replies the staffed and satcheled shaman. The riddles go on in a manner reminiscent of Socrates with one question being answered by posing another.

Intrigued but still annoyed, Simba is engaged. Rational thought and conversation likely would have lost him by now. The priestly monkey shows concern and keeps the stirrings alive; Simba's trouble is soon to become his servant, his wounded past the path to lead him home.

At once, after Simba's dismissive remark to Rafiki concerning the latter's bizarre behavior, Rafiki drops a single truth: *I know who you are; you're Mufasa's boy.* And then the Baboon is off. It is now Simba who chases and desires to know more. It could be nothing but painful to speak of his father, but the gentle, strange monkey has lovingly tugged at that pain. Simba is his; the therapeutic relationship has begun, the pathos entered.

With progressive disclosure in an environment of mystery, Simba tells Rafiki he *could not possibly 'know' his father -- he died.* The shamen: *Wrong again. He is alive, come I show you; you follow old Rafiki, he knows the way.*

The scene which now unfolds is filled with an actual, and highly symbolic, journey through the thick brush and a gnarled path into darkness. Loud drums again mark the lion's clumsey efforts to follow the smaller, more nimble shaman as he makes passage in a way suggesting how it is *he knows the way.* Undoubtedly, Rafiki has made this journey before. Before reaching the small, quiet reflecting pool at the journey's end, Rafiki halts and quiets the adrenaline laden cub. *Shhhhhh* says the Shaman, and then points to the water. *Look there.*

Simba gazes and with softer, reflective music returning; he sees his countenance. Frustration returning, Rafiki points again and encourages Simba: *Look H-a-r-d-e-r.* As Simba gazes more deeply, an image of his father appears. The vision is terrifying, and Simba immediately shouts, asking Mufasa, *Father, why did you leave me?* No real answer is given. Only the thrice given admonition flows from the vision and the mouth of a father who had earlier told his son he would always be with him. *Simba, you are more than you have become. You must take your place in the book of life.* Mufasa evaporates as he appeared, and Rafiki and Simba are out of the cave under a bright moon. It is dark, and there is light.

What was that asks the Shamen of a still quiet and stunned, aware, Simba. Returning to his quizzical posture, Rafiki answers his own question with a *perhaps. Maybe the weather*, he suggests.

For his part, Simba soberly asserts *Whatever it was, it doesn't matter; it's in the past.* Suddenly, a thud. Rafiki's staff strikes the head of the Lion. *Hey, that hurt; why'd you do that ?* Rafiki: It *doesn't matter, it's in the past.*

After Simba grabs the stick, which Rafiki makes very clear is not *just a stick*, and throws it off, the awakened cub begins to run off.

Hey, where are you going? Come back, shouts the Shaman.

I have to go back... I am going home, proclaims Simba. And like a good therapist or priest who realizes he is part of a larger process, Rafiki rejoices even as he acknowledges that he will always welcome Simba back. *Hey, come back; Go on, get out of here.*

Rafiki, like the holy one, has taken initiative and followed Simba's wanderings. Using himself and every other symbol at hand, the shaman invited the young King to *look harder* and become aware that he is more than who he had become. With ritual and mutual story telling, Simba was able to enter the journey, safely guided and directed back home.

The conclusion to which we are led is that rediscovery of soul through the unconscious results in both a theological and religious concern. The former appears when we try to formulate this inner religious life with all its contradictory complexities and to relate it to official dogmas about the nature of God; the latter appears in the reawakened presense of inner myth and sense of destiny, the sense that one is somehow meant. To be meant implies a transcendent power that calls, chooses, or means something with one, a power which gives meaning.

The inner connection to one's life as a ritual and oneself as a symbol of everyman's common humanity remythologizes the course of events, returning numinosity to the mundane. [109]

Chapter Six Notes

[101] Sperry, op. cit., pg. 3
[102] Hillman, op. cit., In Search, pg. 21-22
[103] Ibid. pg. 22
[104] Ashley and O'Rourke, op. cit., pg. 5
[105] Hillman, op. cit., Insearch, pg. 26
[106] Ashley and O'Rourke, op. cit., pg. 6
[107] Hillman, op. cit., In Search, pg. 56
[108] ibid.
[109] Ibid., pg. 59-60

Select Bibliography

Achterberg, Jeanne: *Imagery In Healing* [1985] Shambhala, Boston

Alcoholics Anonymous ("The Big Book") [1984] Alcoholics Anonymous World Services, New York City

Ansbacher, Heinz and Rowena: *The Individual Psychology of Alfred Adler* [1959] Basic Books, Inc., NY

Ashley, Benedict M. & O'Rourke, Kevin D.: *Health Care Ethics* [1982] The Catholic Health Association of the United States, St. Louis, MO.

Atkinson, Donald T.: *Magic, Myth and Medicine* [1956] The World Publishing Company, NY

Campbell, Joseph: *The Hero With a Thousand Faces* [1949] MJF Books, NY

Campbell, Joseph: *The Mythic Image* [1974] Princeton University Press, Princeton NJ

Conn, Joanne Wolski: *Spirituality and Personal Maturity* [1989] Integration/Paulist Press, NY

Corsini, Raymond J. et. al. *Current Psychotherapies* [1979] F. E. Peacock Publishers Inc., Itasca, Illinois

Crowley, Vivianne: *Jungian Spirituality* [1998] Thorsons, Harper Collins Publishers, London

Cunningham, Lawerence: *The Catholic Experience* [1986] Crossroad, New York

Dulles, Avery: *The Priestly Office* [1997] Paulist Press, NY

Dykstra, Craig & Parks, Sharon [ed.]: *Faith Development and Fowler* [1986] Religious Education Press, Birmingham, Alabama

Eliade, Mircea: *Cosmos and History* [1959] Harper Torchbooks/Harper & Row, NY

Eliade, Mircea: *Images and Symbols* [1991] Princeton
University Press, Princeton, NJ

Eliade, Mircea: *Symbolism, the Sacred, and the Arts* [1992]
Continuum, NY

Erikson, Erik: *Childhood and Society* [1963] W W Norton
& Company, NY

Evans, Richard I.: *Carl Rogers* [1975] E P Dutton, New
York

Godin, Andre: *The Psychological Dynamics of Religious
Experience* [1985] Religious Education Press,
Birmingham, Alabama

Griffiths, Bede: *A New Vison of Reality* [1989] Templegate
Publishers, Springfield, Illinos

Groeschel, Benedict J.: *Spiritual Passages* [1992] Crossroad,
NY

Helminiak, David A.: *Religion and the Human Sciences*
[1998] The State University of New York Press,
Albany

Helminiak, David A.: *The Human Core of Spirituality* [1996]
State University of New York, Albany

Hillman, James: *Insearch* [1967] Spring Publications,
Dallas, Texas

Hillman, James: *The Myth of Analysis* [1972] Harper
Perennial/Harper Collins, NY

Hitchcock, John: *The Web of the Universe* [1991] Paulist
Press, NY

Jung, Carl G.: *Memories, Dreams, Reflections* [1963]
Vintage/Random House, NY

Jung, Carl G.: *Modern Man in Search of a Soul* [1933]
Harvest Book/Harcourt Brace & Co., London

Jung, Carl Gustav: *Psychology and Western Religion* [1984]
Princeton University Press

Kelsey, Morton T.: *Prophetic Ministry* [1982] Crossroad,
New York

Leary, Daniel J.: *Voices of Convergence* [1969] The Bruce
Publishing Company, Milwaukee

Leech, Kenneth: *Soul Friend* [1979] Sheldon Press, London

Macquarrie, John: *Paths In Spirituality* [1992] Morehouse Publishing, Harrisburg, PA

Macquarrie, John: *Principles of Christian Theology* [1977] Charles Scribner's Sons, NY

Marty, Martin E. & Vaux, Kenneth L., [ed.]: *Health/Medicine and the Faith Traditions* [1982] Fortress Press, Philadelphia

May, Gerald G.: *Care of Mind, Care of Spirit* [1982] Harper San Fancisco

May, Rollo: *The Art of Counseling* [1967] Abingdon Press, NY

Miller, William R. [ed.]: *Integrating Sprirituality Into Treatment* [1999] American Psychological Association, Washington DC

Moltmann, Jurgen: *Man.* [1971] Fortress Press, Philadelphia

Morgan, John H.: *Being Human* [2002] Quill Books, Cloverdale Corp., Bristol IN.

Morgan, John H.: *From Freud to Frankl* [1987] Wyndham Hall Press

Morgan, John H.: *Scholar, Priest, and Pastor* [1998] GTF Books USA

O Murchu, Diarmund: *Reclaiming Spirituality* [1999] Crossroad, NY

Otto, Rudolf: *The Idea of the Holy* [1967] Oxford University Press, London

Pruyser, Paul: *The Minister As Diagnostician.* [1976] The Westminster Press,   Philadelphia

Reiff, Philip: *The Triumph of the Therapeutic* [1966] Harper & Row, NY

Rogers, Carl R.: *On Becoming A Person* [1961] Houghton Mifflin Company, Boston

Roof, Wade Clark: *A Generation of Seekers* [1994] Harper San Francisco

Smart, Ninian: *Dimensions of the Sacred* [1995] University of California Press, Berkeley CA

Smith, C. Michael: *Jung and Shamanism* [1997] Paulist Press, NY

Sperry, Len: *Transforming Self and Community* [2002] The Liturgical Press Collegeville, Minnesota

Stein, Murray: *Jung's Treatment of Christianity* [1986] Chiron Publications, Illinois

Storr, Anthony: *Freud & Jung* [1989] Oxford University Press

Storr, Anthony: *The Essential Jung* [1993] Princeton University Press, Princeton NJ

Van Gennep, Arnold: *The Rites of Passage* [1960] The University of Chicago Press, Chicago

Vatican Council II The Conciliar and Post Conciliar Documents. [1975] Costello Publishing Company, NY

Wainwright, Geoffrey: *Doxology* [1980] Oxford University Press, New York

Walsh, Roger & Vaughan, Frances [ed.] *Paths Beyond Ego* [1993] Penguin Putnam Inc., NY

Walsh, Roger N.: *The Spirit of Shamanism* [1990] Jeremy P. Tarcher, Inc., Los Angeles

Wexler, Philip: *Mystical Society* [2000] Westview Press, Boulder CO

Whitmont, Edward C.: *The Symbolic Quest* [1960] Princeton University Press, Princeton, NJ

Whitson, Robley Edward: *The Coming Convergence of World Religions* [1992] The United Institute; The Cloverdale Library, Bristol, Indiana

Wilber, Ken: *Integral Psychology* [2000] Shambala, Boston & London

Wolff-Salin, Mary: *No Other Light* [1989] Crossroad, NY

Worgul, George S., Jr.: *From Magic to Metaphor* [1980] Paulist Press, New York

Other Sources

Monitor On Psychology, A Publication of the American
Psychological Association; December 2003; Vol. 34,
NO. 11: Washington, DC

Newsweek Magazine, November 28, 1994, New York, NY;
Special Edition: *The Search for the Sacred, America's Quest
for Spiritual Meaning*